Exercise for Knee and Hip Replacement

Erin Erb Roblero, MSPT, C-PT

DSWFitness   Tucson, Arizona

A special thanks to our course reviewers.

Marlyn Black, BS
Personal Trainer
Pyramid Profiles
Lakeland, FL

Paticia Streit Perez, MS, ATC
President
One Fit Mama
Oreland, PA

Christy Rusdal, MPT
Physical Therapist
St. Peter's Hospital
Helena, MT

Cheri Tatem, BA
Exercise Therapist
Strength Insight
Boulder, CO

Cover Designer: Audra Mitchell
Editor and Text Designer: Karen Thomas

Photography: Daniel Snyder
Model: Susan Bovre

ISBN-13: 978-0-9790787-1-2
ISBN-10: 0-9790787-1-7

Unconditional Guarantee

If you are not completely satisfied with the Desert Southwest Fitness correspondence course *Exercise and Knee and Hip Replacement,* you may exchange your course or receive a full refund, less shipping and handling charges. Materials must be returned unmarked and intact to our office within 30 days of receiving them. All refunds will be made in the same payment method as received.

Copyright

© 2007 by Desert Southwest Fitness, Inc. All rights reserved. No part of this work may be reproduced or transmitted in any form or by any means, electronic or mechanical, including photocopying and recording, or by any information storage or retrieval system, except as may be expressly permitted by the 1976 Copyright Act or in writing by the publisher.

Disclaimer

This learning guide is informational only. The data and information contained herein are based upon information from various published as well as unpublished sources and merely represent general training, exercise, and health literature and practices as summarized by the authors and editors. Care has been taken to confirm the accuracy of the information presented and to describe generally accepted practice. However, the author and publisher are not responsible for errors or omissions or for any consequences from application of the information in this workbook. The publisher of this learning guide makes no guarantees or warranties, express or implied, regarding the currentness, completeness, or scientific accuracy of this information, nor does the publisher guarantee or warrant the fitness, marketability, efficacy, or accuracy of this information for any particular purpose. This summary of information from unpublished sources, books, research journals, and articles is not intended to replace the advice or attention of medical or healthcare professionals. This summary is also not intended to direct anyone's behavior or replace anyone's independent professional judgment. If you have a problem with your health, before you embark on any health, fitness, or sports training program, including the programs herein, please seek advice and clearance from a qualified medical or healthcare professional. The publishers have made every effort to trace the copyright holders for borrowed material. If they have inadvertently overlooked any, they will be pleased to make necessary arrangements at the first opportunity.

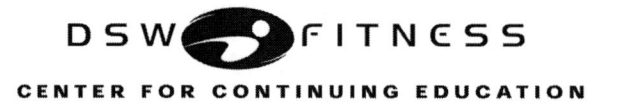

DSW FITNESS
CENTER FOR CONTINUING EDUCATION

602 E. ROGER RD • TUCSON, AZ 85705 • 520.292.0011 • FAX 520.292.0066 • EXAMS@DSWFITNESS.COM • WWW.DSWFITNESS.COM

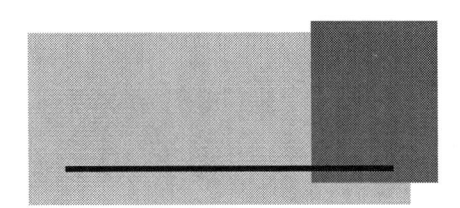

Contents

1 Introduction to Total Joint Replacement 1
Joint Anatomy 2
Joint Classification 2
Synovial Joints 4
Osteoarthritis 6
Other Conditions Leading to Total Joint Replacement 9
Prosthesis 11
Fixation: Cement Versus Cementless 11
Hip Replacement Technique 12
Knee Replacement Technique 15
Alternative Techniques and Recent Improvements 17
Study Questions 19

2 Recovery 21
Physical Therapy and Exercise 21
Complications 22
Role of the Fitness Trainer 25
Study Questions 30

3 Health Screening and Client Assessment 31
Health Screening for Physical Activity 31
Client Assessment 38
Study Questions 46

4 Exercises 47
Total Knee Replacement Exercises 47
Total Hip Replacement Exercises 62
Study Questions 78

5 Case Studies 79
Total Knee Replacement 79
Total Hip Replacement 82

Answer Keys 85

References 87

About the Author 89

CHAPTER 1

Introduction to Total Joint Replacement

A joint replacement surgery consists of removing a damaged joint and replacing it with a prosthesis, or an artificial joint, made from metal alloys, high-grade plastic, and cement. The two goals of a joint replacement are (1) to improve function and (2) decrease pain. Prior to the surgery, it may be difficult for the person to walk, climb stairs, bathe, and get in and out of a chair. The intent of the surgery is to return the person to a more active and independent lifestyle, thereby improving the person's quality of life. A total joint replacement is usually considered after all other options and treatments have been used to manage the person's pain and disability. These other options may have included medication, physical therapy, and activity modification.

A total joint replacement is also known as a total joint arthroplasty. *Arthro* means joint, and *plasty* means molding or forming surgically. Together, the word *arthroplasty* means the creation of an artificial joint. A British orthopedist, Sir John Charnley, is credited with performing the first total hip replacement in 1962. Today, over 760,000 Americans undergo joint replacement surgery in one form or another each year (AAOS Department of Research and Scientific Affairs, 2002). According to the American Academy of Orthopedic Surgeons, 400,000 of the surgeries in 2002 were knee replacements and 343,000 were hip replacements (AAOS Department of Research and Scientific Affairs, 2002). Although hip and knee joints are the most common joints to be replaced, other joints such as the shoulder, ankle, toe, and even finger are replaced with good results.

With advances in the design and construction of artificial joints, the number of joint replacements performed each year continues to increase and have higher success rates in the long term. According to the American Academy of Orthopedic Surgeons, a hip or knee replacement can last 20 years in 80% of the people who undergo the surgery (Bren, 2004).

Joint replacement surgery was once considered only for the elderly or inactive. Although most people who undergo joint replacements are between the ages of 60 and 80, individuals are evaluated on a case-by-case basis, and it is not uncommon for a younger person to have a joint replacement surgery. The decision to undergo a joint replacement must be made with careful consideration of the possible risks and benefits of the surgery. A medical doctor who possesses the appropriate knowledge of the surgery should help guide the person through the decision-making process.

Joint Anatomy

A joint is made of two or more bones that come together and are connected by strong fibrous tissue. The joint allows smooth movement to occur between the bones and absorbs the shock from repetitive movements. Joints are made to withstand repeated movements in an efficient and smooth manner. When one portion of the joint does not function properly, the joint itself has difficulty performing its job. This occurs with conditions such as osteoarthritis in which the cartilage in the joint starts to wear down.

Joint Classification

Joints are classified by the way one bone articulates with the other and the type of movement they allow. One example is the ball-and-socket joint. In this type of joint, the end of one bone is round like a ball, while the surface of the other bone is hollow. This allows the convex, or rounded, portion of the ball to fit closely within the concave depression of the other bone.

Figure 1. Shoulder ball-and-socket joint

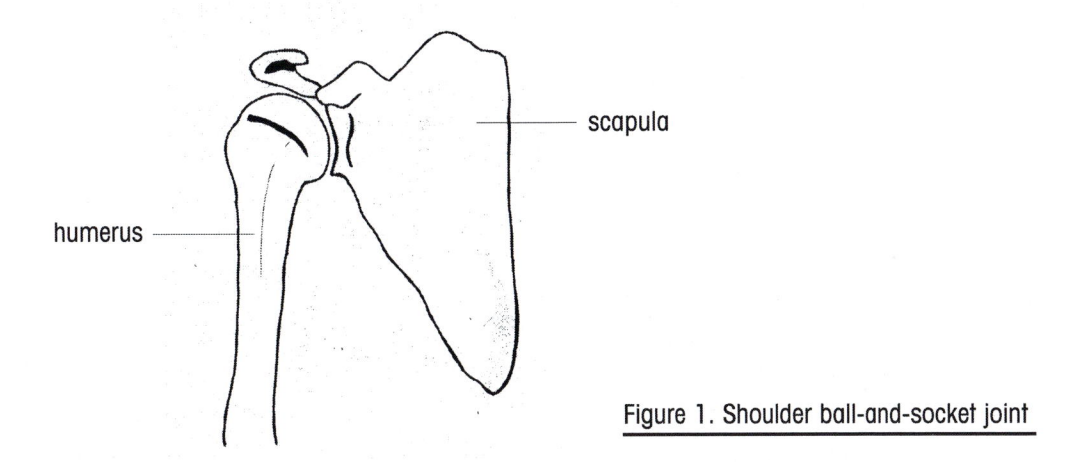

The shoulder joint is an example of a ball-and-socket joint. The long bone in the upper arm, the humerus, articulates with the shallow portion of the scapula called the glenoid fossa. The rounded head of the humerus is the ball and the hollowed-out portion of the scapula is the socket.

In the case of the shoulder, many motions are possible, including circumduction, flexion, extension, abduction, adduction, internal rotation, and external rotation. The hip joint is another example of a ball-and-socket joint. The head of the long thigh bone, or femur, joins together with the shallow portion of the pelvis called the acetabulum. Of all the different joints, the ball-and-socket joint has the capacity for the greatest amount of movement.

Another type of joint is the hinge joint. In this type of joint, a convex bone surface fits into the concave portion of another bone. Like a hinge on a door, this joint allows only one plane of motion: flexion and extension. The knee is an example of a hinge joint.

Synovial Joints

Both the ball-and-socket and hinge joints are examples of synovial joints. All freely moving, or synovial joints, have certain characteristics in common.

On either end of the bones a smooth layer of cartilage allows the joint to move freely and without pain. Cartilage is a slippery protein coating on the ends of each bone serving as cushioning and shock absorption. Cartilage is composed of 65% to 85% water along with three other substances: collagen, proteoglycans, and chondrocytes. Collagen is the building block of connective tissues. Proteoglycans combine with collagen to form a tissue that allows the cartilage to be flexible and absorb shock. The chondrocytes assist the cartilage in growing and staying healthy.

Covering the outside of the joint is a strong membranous capsule that keeps the bones in close approximation. Inside the capsule, a smooth, thin lining called the synovium secretes fluid to reduce friction and degeneration inside the joint. Synovial fluid lubricates the joint and is a source of nutrition for the cartilage.

Figure 2 shows the two vertically positioned bones that have plenty of space separating them along with adequate cartilage (black shading) on the ends of each bone. The outside line represents the joint capsule, and the striated inner line represents the synovium. The grey-shaded area between the ends of the bones is representative of the synovial fluid.

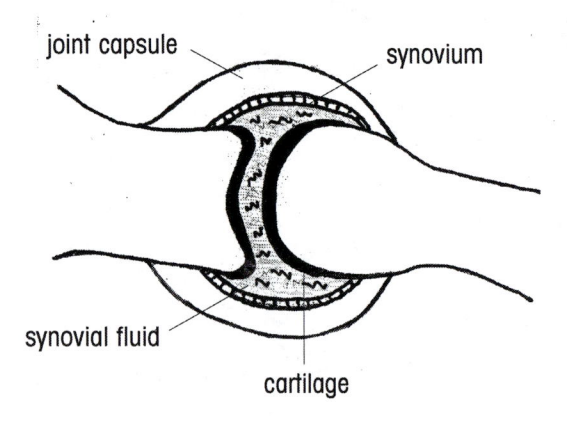

Figure 2. Normal joint

Figure 3. Knee joint and ligaments

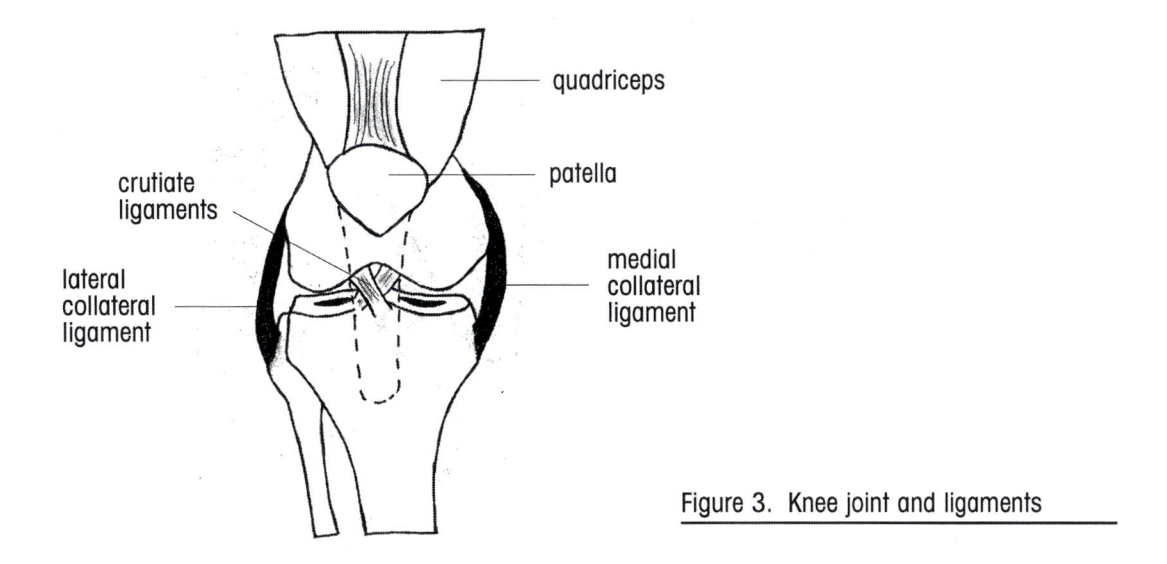

The other structures that keep the joint stable include ligaments, tendons, and muscles. Ligaments are tough tissue connecting one bone to another, and tendons connect muscle to bone. Muscles are strong bands of tissue that contract and produce movement in the joint. Together the ligaments, tendons, and muscles stabilize the joint and allow it to move through its full range of motion.

As an example, the knee joint has a number of muscles, ligaments, and tendons that help stabilize it and keep the knee functioning safely and properly. The anterior and posterior cruciate ligaments are located inside the capsule and prevent excess rotation of the knee. The medial and lateral collateral ligaments run along either side of the knee joint to prevent excess side-bending stress.

In addition to other musculature, the quadriceps extend the knee, and the hamstrings are responsible for flexing it. With all the components of the joint working properly, a smooth and fluid motion between the bones can be accomplished.

Osteoarthritis

Osteoarthritis is a degenerative joint disease that causes destruction of a joint, resulting in pain and impaired movement. In the US, 20 million people suffer from this disease. According to the National Institute of Arthritis and Musculoskeletal and Skin Diseases (NIAMS), osteoarthritis is the most common reason for having a hip or knee replacement (www.naims.nih.gov, 2002). Osteoarthritis is a leading cause of disability in adults. It is most common in the knees, hips, fingers, thumbs, lower back, and neck. There are no definite answers for what causes the disease, but researchers believe that it includes a number of factors, including joint stress, previous injury, the aging process, and being overweight. Most often, osteoarthritis comes on slowly. Early symptoms may include joint aching after physical exercise. Osteoarthritis has signs and symptoms that are easily recognizable.

> **Osteoarthritis Warning Signs**
> * Pain in the joint—intermittent or constant, often worse at the end of the day, dull and aching quality or occasionally sharp.
> * Pain that is progressive in nature—has gotten worse over time, increases with greater activity levels.
> * Stiffness in a joint or limitations in joint movement, especially after sitting or lying down for a long period of time.
> * Swelling around the joint.
> * Possible crunching or creaking sounds with joint movement.

Disease Progression

As people age or are injured, the cartilage that once served as a protective cushion between the two bones of a joint begins to wear away. As the cartilage wears away with repetitive motion of the joint, the two bones begin to rub against one another, causing inflammation and pain. Pain can lead to limited joint range of

Introduction to Total Joint Replacement   7

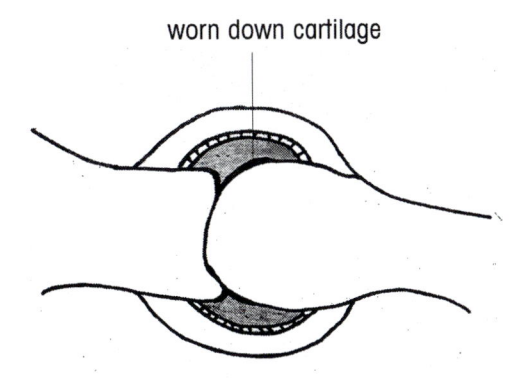

worn down cartilage

Figure 4. Arthritic joint.

motion and decreased activity. A combination of factors including pressure on the nerve endings, muscle tension, and fatigue can cause the sensation of pain. In response to the decrease in movement and overall mobility, the muscles in the lower extremity weaken, resulting in overall body deconditioning.

Figure 4 shows two bones that are rubbing together and have very little cartilage at their ends.

Bone spurs, or osteophytes, can develop around the edges of the joint in response to the ends of the bones rubbing together. Cartilage and even small pieces of bone can break away and float inside the joint, leading to even greater damage and pain.

Progression of Osteoarthritis
1. Cartilage degeneration
2. Pain and inflammation (possible bone spur formation)
3. Limited joint range of motion and decreased activity level
4. Weakened lower body muscles
5. Body deconditioning and decreased mobility

Diagnosis

A physician uses a combination of methods to rule out or diagnose osteoarthritis. These include a medical history, description of the symptoms, physical examination, x-rays, and possibly blood tests to rule out other conditions. Once osteoarthritis is diagnosed, a number of treatments can be utilized.

Treatment

Exercise

Exercise can include physical therapy, occupational therapy, or personal training. Exercise increases the strength of the muscles that support the joint, increases flexibility, reduces body weight, improves psychological well-being, and decreases pain. Types of exercise include:

- **Strength training** Using low weights with multiple repetitions helps improve muscular strength and joint stability, which is important for a return to functional activities.
- **Aerobic activities** Exercises such as walking or biking raise the heart rate and can improve function of the circulatory and respiratory systems.
- **Flexibility training** Stretching can help improve joint range of motion and ease movement.

Weight Control

Losing excess body weight will reduce the stress placed on weight-bearing joints like the hip and knee. A healthy diet and regular exercise can help regulate an appropriate weight.

Medications

The physician may prescribe anti-inflammatories or other pain-relieving drugs. These include:

- Acetaminophen—a pain reliever that does not reduce inflammation and is unlikely to cause stomach irritation (Tylenol).

- NSAIDs (nonsteroidal anti-inflammatory drugs)—medications used to decrease inflammation and pain (Advil, Aleve, Motrin).
- Topical creams, sprays, or rubs.
- Mild narcotics.
- Corticosteroids injections.

Rest and Activity Modification
Avoiding overexertion and resting the joints between performing daily tasks can ease the stress placed on the joint surfaces.

Pain Control
Moist heat, ice, hydrotherapy in a warm pool, knee braces or splints, walking aids such as a cane or walker, acupuncture, or nutritional supplements can help control and relieve painful symptoms.

Surgery
Surgery is usually used as the last resort when a person is unable to attain pain relief through the above methods and has severe limitations in functional activities such as walking, bathing, toileting, and getting in and out of bed or a chair. Before surgery, the physician will look closely at the client's general health, weight, age, joint alignment, bone density, and nutrition. If the client is young, the prosthesis may wear out faster than it would in a less active person. Osteoporosis or stress fractures need to be treated first because the prosthesis requires good anchorage to keep it in place. Orthoscopic surgery is a less invasive surgery that is sometimes an option before resorting to total joint replacement.

Other Conditions Leading to Total Joint Replacement

Osteoarthritis is the primary cause of joint deterioration that requires a total joint replacement. The following are other medical conditions that may necessitate the surgery.

Rheumatoid Arthritis (RA)

RA is a systemic autoimmune disease characterized by inflammation and thickening of the joint space. This chronic condition can lead to cartilage loss, pain, and stiffness.

Post-Traumatic Arthritis

Previous bony fracture or ligament tears from injury can lead to the early degeneration of a joint, as well as pain and limitations in movement.

Hip Fracture

A hip may need to be replaced if fixing the fracture is not possible. One possible cause of a fractured hip is a fall.

Hip Necrosis

Necrosis is the death of the bony matrix that can occur from a hip fracture, use of certain drugs, and other diseases or disorders that cause a disruption of the blood flow to the head of the femur. Without a viable blood supply, the bone dies and necrosis occurs.

Reasons to Consider a Total Joint Replacement

* Severe pain that interferes with everyday activities.
* Pain during rest.
* Chronic swelling that does not improve with activity modification or medications.
* Deformity or stiffness which limits joint range of motion.
* Inadequate pain relief from medications such as NSAIDs.
* Failure to improve with other treatments such as physical therapy, cortisone injections, or other surgical procedures.

Prosthesis

The prosthesis, or artificial joint, is inserted into the body to replace the damaged portion of the joint. The prosthesis is designed to function just like a normal joint. Because prostheses are medical devices, they are regulated in the United States by the Food and Drug Administration (FDA) and must be approved for safety and effectiveness. Currently, the FDA has approximately 750 approved designs on file for hip replacement prostheses alone. Whether the prosthesis is used for a hip, knee, or shoulder replacement, all the materials have these things in common:

- They are biocompatible and will not trigger a rejection response within the body.
- They resist degradation and corrosion so the strength and shape of the prosthesis will not be compromised over a long period of time. The components are designed to resist wear and tear so proper joint function can be maintained.
- They have similar characteristics of the structures they replaced. For example, the prosthesis is both flexible and strong enough to withstand the pressure of weight-bearing loads. Furthermore, the components move smoothly against one other, minimizing the amount of microscopic debris generated within the joint.

Fixation: Cement versus Cementless

One very important consideration for the surgeon is whether to cement the prosthesis into place with a special kind of adhesive. The decision to cement the prosthesis in place is based on a number of factors such as age, weight, quality of the bone, and activity level of the patient.

Designs introduced in 1977 made it possible for the implant to attach directly to the bone without using cement. The porous texture around the implant allows the bone to actually grow into the surface of the prosthesis. Cementless procedures require a longer recovery time because bone growth is essential for the prosthesis to be stable. Six to twelve weeks of partial weight bearing on the affected limb is usually needed for the bone to attach itself to the prosthesis. Strong prosthesis-to-bone bonding is one of the most significant benefits of the cementless procedure; therefore, this type of fixation is often used with younger patients and those who are more active. The cementless technique can be used in both a hip and knee joint replacement.

On the other hand, one of the advantages of a cemented-joint procedure is the ability to put full weight on the leg and walk on it almost immediately. This can translate to quicker rehabilitation. A person who is not able to maintain partial weight-bearing on the operated leg may benefit from the cemented fixation.

An acrylic polymer called polymethylmethacrylate (PMMA) is the most commonly used bone cement. Imagine a caulking gun used in your house to seal the edges of your bathtub. When the caulk is first squeezed out of the tube it is soft and malleable like dough. After 10 to 15 minutes the cement hardens into a solid substance, filling the crevices and acting as a strong sealer. One disadvantage of this type of fixation is the possibility of the cement loosening around the prosthesis over time.

For all the implants, the prosthetic stem and the cavity within the bone must fit together precisely, since new bone growth cannot bridge gaps larger than 1 to 2 mm. Unfortunately, both the cemented and cementless total joint replacements run the risk of loosening, especially if the essential bond between the bone and prosthetic stem is not achieved.

Hip Replacement Technique

The first total hip replacement in the United States was performed around 1969. Today, this operation has become fairly routine. In 2002, 343,000 total hip replacement surgeries were performed. It is estimated that 80% of the hip replacements will last 20 years or more (Bren, 2004).

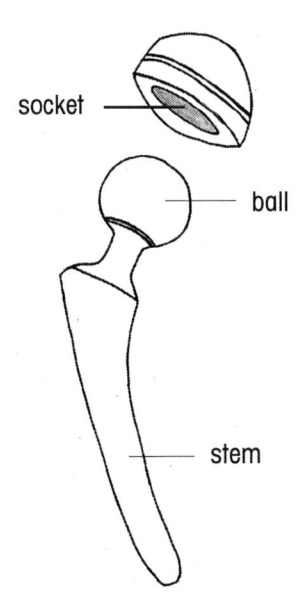

Figure 5. Socket, ball, and stem of a hip replacement

Basic Anatomy

The head of the femur articulates with the shallow portion of the lateral hip called the acetabulum. The gluteus medius, minimus, and maximus muscles all attach at points around the hip joint. There are also smaller hip rotator muscles that are usually cut during the surgery to expose the hip joint. The hip joint capsule keeps the head of the femur within the socket of the acetabulum.

Prosthetic Components of a Total Hip Replacement

A hip prosthesis has three basic parts:

(1) The stem fits into the long bone and provides stability. This prosthetic component is made of metal such as stainless steel, alloys of cobalt, and chrome, as well as titanium. In figure 5, the stem is the longest part of the prosthesis.

(2) The ball is a rounded sphere on the end of the stem. It is made of either a cobalt/chromium mixture or ceramic materials (aluminum

oxide or zirconium oxide) polished smooth to allow the maximum amount of rotation within the socket. The stem and ball are one piece in most designs, but they can also come separately to allow for a more customized fit.

(3) The socket is fit into the hollow area on the side of the hip bone. It is made of either durable high-density polyethylene, metal, or a combination of polyethylene backed by metal. The grey-shaded area in figure 5 (previous page) is where the ball is inserted into the socket.

Surgical Steps

There are a number of different surgical approaches. The two used most often are the posterior and the lateral approach. The muscles that are cut or disrupted during the procedure depend on the type of approach the surgeon uses. For instance, with the lateral approach, an incision is made on the outside of the thigh. The gluteus medius and the vastus lateralis muscles may be split to allow for the hip capsule to be visualized. With the posterior approach, the gluteus maximus tendon is cut and the quadratus femoris may need to be released if the surgeon requires greater exposure to the hip. It is also important for the surgeon to protect the sciatic nerve that runs through the gluteal area. Once cut, the deep hip rotator muscles are sometimes peeled back to provide a layer of protection to the sciatic nerve during the remainder of the surgery.

After the muscles are cut or separated, the femoral head is removed or dislocated from the socket so the joint cavity opens. The acetabulum is cleaned of damaged cartilage and bone. A special tool is used to smooth and enlarge the surface of the socket to prepare it for the cup-like component to be inserted. The prosthetic shell is placed securely within the prepared socket and may be held in place by the use of cement or screws.

The femoral head is sawed off and a cavity, or hollowed-out space, is created within the femur that will match the shape of the stem. The stem and ball portion of the prosthesis is inserted into the femur and may be held in place by the use of cement. The incision is closed after the ball is placed within the shallow area and the joint is aligned correctly.

Knee Replacement Technique

The knee is the largest joint in the body. It is called a hinge joint because it bends and straightens like a hinge on a door. This is a simplified image because the knee joint is really a combination of three bones (femur, tibia, and patella) coming together with rotation occurring within the joint.

The first knee replacement was performed around 1968. Today, over 400,000 knee replacement surgeries are performed each year in the US. Studies have shown that a total knee replacement has a 95% chance of lasting 15 to 20 years (aaos.org, 2005).

Basic Anatomy

The lower end of the femur, or the medial and lateral condyles, rotate on the tibia. The tibia's upper portion is like a shallow shelf where the condyles sit. A thick cartilaginous disc called the meniscus sits between the two bones to absorb shock, reduce friction, and increase the conformity between the femur and tibia. The patella, or knee cap, slides in the groove on the top of the femur when the joint bends and straightens. The quadriceps and the hamstrings surround the joint and give it strength for weight-bearing activities. The anterior and posterior cruciate ligaments, along with the collateral ligaments, give the knee stability both inside as well as outside the joint capsule, respectively.

Prosthetic Components of a Total Knee Replacement

A knee prosthesis has three components:

(1) The femoral component covers the end of the femur and wraps

Figure 6. Femoral, tibial, and patellar components of a knee replacement

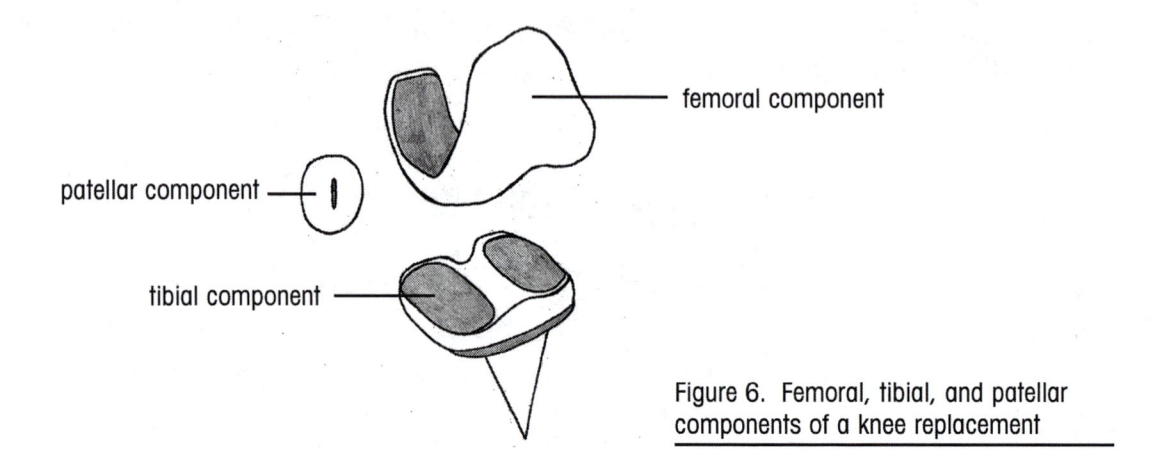

around the medial and lateral condyles.

(2) The tibial component attaches to the plateau, or upper portion of the tibia. It has two indentations where the femoral component glides and rotates, allowing the knee to bend and straighten.

(3) The patellar component covers the underside of the kneecap. Depending on the condition of the patella, this component does not always need to be replaced.

Surgical Steps

A 6- to 12-inch incision is made lengthwise down the front of the thigh. The quadriceps muscle is moved out of the way to expose the knee joint. Specialized instruments remove the damaged ends of the tibia and femur. A metal component is fitted on the femur and a plastic component is placed on the tibia. If the patella is also arthritic, the underside is cut flat and replaced with another plastic component.

During both the knee and hip replacement surgeries, the person's lower extremity is brought through the full range of motion while they are still under anesthesia to make sure the components glide smoothly and to ensure the patient has full joint mobility.

Alternative Techniques and Recent Improvements

Since the introduction of joint replacements in the 1960s, new techniques for inserting the prostheses have been developed. Improvements to the prosthetic design and the materials used to make them have had a positive impact on prosthetic durability and the long-term success rate of the joint replacement.

Minimally Invasive

One of the most recent advancements in joint replacement is the minimally invasive surgery that refers to the size of surgical incision. In a normal hip replacement, a 10- to 12-inch incision would be made to expose the area. In a minimally invasive surgery, either one 4-inch cut or two 2-inch cuts are made. Likewise, for a knee replacement, the typical 6- to 12-inch incision would be 4 to 5 inches long instead.

Reported benefits of this type of surgery include decreased bleeding from the incision, decreased trauma to the muscles and tendons, and decreased pain, leading to improved rehabilitation capacity. A potential drawback of the surgery is it is more difficult to perform than the traditional joint replacement, which means more time on the operating table, thereby, increasing the risk of infection. This procedure also requires the use of x-rays to fit the implant into the proper position. Because the joint is less exposed during the minimally invasive surgery, it requires around 2 to 3 more hours to complete than the traditional surgery.

The minimally invasive procedure uses the same implants as the traditional joint replacement, but specially designed instruments are needed to prepare the joint and place the implants properly. Because this surgery is relatively new, another 10 to 15 years is needed to judge its effectiveness and long-term success rate.

Hemiarthroplasty

With this surgery, only one portion of the damaged portion of the joint is replaced. Microscopic debris caused by wear and tear between the two surfaces is minimized when only one part of the joint is artificial. Usually it is the head of the femur that is replaced by a prosthesis, while the joint socket remains untouched. Hemiarthroplastys are often used with hip fractures and can be performed on someone with avascular necrosis if there is any remaining articular cartilage on the acetabulum.

Other Procedures

Other types of joint replacement are performed less frequently. Metal-on-metal joints have both components made of metal but few of these prostheses are FDA approved. Ceramic-on-ceramic prostheses are thought to withstand the wear and tear of people with more active lifestyles, but this type of prosthesis has not been on the market long enough to have any long-term studies regarding their effectiveness. Another new technique is called a partial-knee replacement. In this surgery only one of the damaged knee condyles is replaced. This can be performed with a minimally invasive procedure. Initial studies show that 95% of these implants are functioning well after 15 years.

Another technique involves a knee replacement that not only moves forward and backward, but also has a small amount of rotation inward and outward. This "rotating" knee replacement is thought to more accurately represent the knee joint. Some practitioners believe this type of knee replacement will last longer because the extra motion acts more like a normal knee joint, while others argue that the extra movement will cause the prosthesis to wear out faster. No one can know for certain until the prosthesis has been on the market longer and studies of the long-term results become available.

Study Questions

Complete the following questions. The answer key is on page 85.

1. Name the two primary goals of a joint replacement surgery.

    (1) _improve function_

    (2) _decrease pain_

2. True or false. The word arthroplasty means the creation of an artificial joint.

3. List three warning signs of osteoarthritis.

    (1) _Pain in the joint_

    (2) _Stiffness + ROM reduction_

    (3) _Swelling_

4. True or false. Osteoarthritis is the leading cause of disability in adults.

5. True or false. Surgery is usually performed as the last resort after trying other treatment options.

6. Name three conditions that may necessitate a total joint replacement.

    (1) _Severe pain, interfering w/ daily activities_

    (2) _Pain during rest_

    (3) _Chronic swelling_

    (4) _Deformation or stiffness_

    (5) _other methods failed_

7. List three reasons a client may want to consider having a total joint replacement.

    (1) _Quality of life_

    (2) _Pain cannot be managed by Meds_

    (3) _Failure to improve w/ other treatments_

8. Name the three components of a hip joint prosthesis.

    (1) _Socket_

    (2) _Ball_

    (3) _Stem_

9. True or <u>false</u>. In a cemented joint replacement procedure, the bone grows into the prosthesis.

10. <u>True</u> or false. An advantage to using the cemented procedure is the ability to put full weight on the leg almost immediately.

11. List three benefits of minimally invasive joint replacement surgery.

    (1) _decreased bleeding_

    (2) _decreased pain_

    (3) _decreased trauma to muscles + tendons_

CHAPTER 2

Recovery

Recovery from a total joint replacement can last anywhere from a few weeks to a few months. Recovery usually begins in the hospital the day after surgery. Once the patient is medically stable, he or she begins their recovery process by walking with a walker or crutches and performing exercises in his or her room.

Physical Therapy and Exercise

Two initial goals of physical therapy are (1) to prevent contracture or tightening of the muscles surrounding the joint and (2) to assist the client in increasing muscle strength for joint stability. Most importantly, physical therapy helps the patient to perform activities of daily living, like walking.

The decision of which assistive device the patient should use for walking is determined by the physician and the physical therapist. The choice of device also depends on how much weight the client is allowed to put on the leg. If the patient is not allowed to bear weight on the leg, a walker is used. Crutches can also be used if the patient has good balance. As the patient progresses, a cane can be used in the hand on the opposite side of the surgery, so that weight is transferred away from the involved leg.

The patient can stay in the hospital anywhere from a few days to a couple of weeks depending on his or her medical status and progress with physical therapy. Upon leaving the hospital, the patient may be discharged home or transferred to an inpatient rehabilitation unit where the patient will continue to work on his or her strength, range of motion, and functional activities, such as walking. If the patient is discharged home, physical therapy can be ordered by the physician to be performed at the patient's home. Another option is outpatient physical therapy that can be provided two to three times a week for a month or two. Physical therapy on an outpatient basis is a good transition from exercising at home during the initial recovery and exercising independently at a gym or health club.

Each person recovers from surgery at a different rate depending on age, current physical condition, and medical history.

Complications

Total joint replacements are extremely successful in most people. Nonetheless, complications do occur and may include the following conditions.

Blood Clots

Blood can pool in the lower extremities due to decreased activity. Pain, swelling, and redness in the calves or thighs are indications of blood clots. Anticoagulants or blood thinners are sometimes prescribed to decrease the chance of blood clots. Elastic stockings also help to prevent blood clots. These compression garments come in knee or thigh-high lengths and are worn like pantyhose. Exercise also combats blood clots by improving circulation in the legs.

Infection

Infection can occur at the surgical site or around the prosthesis. It may present in the hospital, after discharge, or a few years later. Other infections within the body may travel through the blood stream to the site of the joint replacement. If an infection is severe enough, the prosthesis may need to be removed. Warning signs of infection include fever, abnormal redness or warmth around the joint, persistent swelling, and unusual pain with activity or rest.

A joint that has been replaced will always be at risk for infection when any invasive procedure is performed. Therefore, clients should always notify their doctor or dentist before invasive procedures are performed. Antibiotics are usually given before, during, and after the procedure in order to prevent infection.

Loosening

One of the major long-term complications of a total joint replacement is the loosening of the prosthesis within the bone. Over time or with excessive wear, cracks in the prosthetic cement can occur and cause the prosthetic stem to become unstable. The prosthesis may then loosen within the bone, causing an increase in pain. Particles from the cement may result in an inflammatory response, which causes cells to remove bits of bone around the implant, leading to further instability. This may occur in those who are overweight or very active, both of which may increase excessive wear on the prosthesis. The risk of prosthetic loosening increases over time.

Dislocation

Dislocation of the hip is more common than dislocation of other joint prostheses. A dislocation occurs when the ball portion of the prosthesis dislodges from the socket. In the very early stages of the total hip replacement recovery it is extremely important for clients to follow hip precautions so they will not dislocate their hip. The precautions include not crossing the legs, not sitting on low chairs or toilets, and not bending at the waist greater than a 90-degree angle. Most hip dislocations can be treated without surgery. Although hip dislocation is more common during the earlier stages of recovery, a risk continues throughout the lifespan of the replacement, especially if the muscles surrounding the hip are not strong. Strengthening exercises for hip stability are important for this reason.

Nerve Injury

Nerve injury is infrequent and often improves over time when it does occur. Nerve injury may occur as a result of the surgical procedure itself and may present as numbness, tingling, or pain in the affected area. These symptoms are common after surgery even without nerve damage, so severe injury to a nerve may not be diagnosed until later in the recovery process. Fortunately, injured nerves in the peripheral nervous system are capable of slow regeneration.

Prosthetic Breakage

Breaking of the prosthesis is a rare occurrence that requires revision surgery. This may happen if the patient has a serious fall or accident that causes damage to the prosthesis itself.

Leg-Length Discrepancy

Leg-length discrepancy can be caused by a slight difference in the length of the prosthesis that is placed into the hip or knee. Occasionally the affected leg may be longer or shorter than the normal one after surgery is completed. A ¼ inch difference in leg length rarely causes problems. Unequal leg lengths of more than a ¼ inch can cause pain in the feet, knees, hips, and back due to uneven pressure on the legs. To equalize the length of the legs, a shoe lift may be needed to avoid hip, knee, or back pain.

Total Joint Revision

If loosening of an implant occurs and presents problems with pain and disability, a total joint revision may be performed. Loosening of the hip or knee implant results from bone loss that occurs from wear on the joint. During normal movement of the joint, the two surfaces of the joint rub against each other and create microscopic particles of debris. The body tries to remove this debris using an inflammatory response. An inflammatory response causes cells to remove bits of bone around the implant, a condition called osteolysis. As wear continues, bone loss increases, along with a greater probability of the implant loosening.

In a joint revision surgery, any or all of the prosthetic components can be replaced. Revision can also be performed due to fracture or other complications. In general, the revision may or may not be a more complicated surgery than the first, but recovery can be more difficult, and the results are generally not as good as the original operation. After a hip revision surgery, hip precautions need to be followed again.

Role of the Fitness Trainer

The fitness professional may start to work with a joint-replacement client when it has been recommended or cleared by a physician or physical therapist. If a client comes to you on his or her own, it is best to contact the physician to ensure that personal training is appropriate for the client at that time. The primary role of the fitness professional is to assist the client to regain lower body strength as well as total body strength, to design an exercise program with activities appropriate for a client with a hip or knee replacement, to improve the client's gait, range of motion, and balance, to monitor precautions and contraindications, and to progress the client to full recovery and a lifestyle of physical activity. If the client has any increased pain or new symptoms relating to the joint, the client should consult his or her physician before continuing with the training routine.

Muscle Training

All joint-replacement patients are strongly encouraged to continue regular exercise and to stay active the rest of their lives. If the muscles are allowed to weaken from inactivity, the patient is at increased risk of falling. According to the American Association of Orthopedic Surgeons, falls are the leading cause of repeat joint replacement surgeries (aaos.org, 2004).

One of the most important aspects of recovery is regaining strength in the lower body. The muscles around the surgery site are weakened from both the lack of activity prior to the surgery and from the incisions that have disrupted the muscle's integrity. Muscle strength in the lower extremity will increase as the exercise program progresses in the following days and weeks.

A study published in 2005 (Mizner et. al) has shown that 1 month after a total knee replacement, quadriceps strength in the involved leg decreased by 62% compared with pre-operative testing. This strength deficit was explained by a combination of muscle atrophy and a decrease in voluntary muscle activation. This study suggests that exercise programs that facilitate voluntary activation may help to counter large strength deficits of the quadriceps following a total knee replacement.

Appropriate Activities and Risk Factors

When a client first comes to see you after joint replacement surgery and physical therapy, it is important to be aware of the type and frequency of activity he or she has been performing. The wear and tear on joint replacements of the hip and knee are similar to the wear and tear on tires. The time it takes to wear out a set of tires depends on how often the car is driven, the terrain it is driven on, how heavy the vehicle is, and whether or not the car is properly maintained. Similarly, the client should be aware of his or her activity level, weight, and physical condition. Making clients aware of these important factors is one way in which personal trainers can help to keep their clients safe and assist their clients in keeping their new joints functioning properly for a long time.

Low-impact activities are the most appropriate for the client with a joint replacement. Activities include walking, swimming, golfing (with spikeless shoes and a cart), bicycling (on level surfaces), stationary bike riding, and ballroom dancing. Activities that put the joint at increased risk of injury are jogging, skiing, horseback riding, tennis (or other racquet sports such as badminton or squash), high-impact aerobics, and contact sports. Long periods of stepping or climbing stairs (stair climber) should be avoided as well. Although most clients would not have been participating in these contraindicated sports to begin with due to pain, some may feel so good after their surgery that they may feel motivated to try these activities.

You may also observe that it is easier for clients to manage their weight after surgery once their pain has decreased, making it easier to exercise. Normal levels of activity should not damage the prosthesis. Regular exercise increases muscular strength, flexibility, and bone density, improves endurance, and heightens self-esteem. So, the joint replacement client has all the reasons in the world to begin or continue an exercise routine.

In a study published in June 2005, researchers at Duke University Medical Center determined that Americans with diabetes, hypertension, and obesity are significantly more likely to suffer from postoperative complications after a major joint replacement surgery (Merritt, 2005). Of these three risk factors, obesity seems to pose the greatest danger for complications. Personal trainers armed with this information can help educate their clients about these conditions and their impact on postoperative joint replacement health.

Activity Level

Weight-Bearing Status
Always ask your client what his or her current weight-bearing status is. If the client is full weight bearing, then find out how long he or she has been allowed to put full weight on the leg. If this change in weight-bearing status was recent, the training routine should not be as advanced as for a client who has been full weight bearing since the day after surgery.

Hip Precautions
Certain movements are prohibited with a client who has had a total hip replacement until his or her physician says the movements are safe to perform. These movements are called hip precautions and help the client avoid dislocation of their hip. The patient may need to follow the hip precautions for 2 to 3 months

or indefinitely, depending on what the surgeon orders. Always ask clients if they are still following hip precautions. Some doctors will have their patients follow the precautions forever, so when in doubt, follow the precautions and follow up with the physician. The following are hip precautions.

Limit hip bending to 90 degrees.

- Keep knees below the hips when seated.
- Don't sit in low chairs or on low toilet seats that raise the knees higher than the hips.
- Don't lean forward while sitting, tying shoes, or putting on socks.
- A device called a reacher can be purchased to help with these activities.
- Don't bend over all the way to pick something off the floor. Use a reacher, bend the knees, or ask someone for help.
- Don't reach down to pull up blankets when lying in bed.
- Use a reacher or keep the covers by your knees.

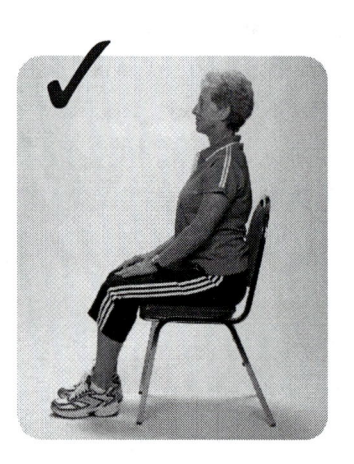

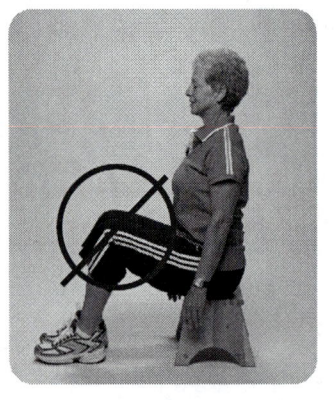

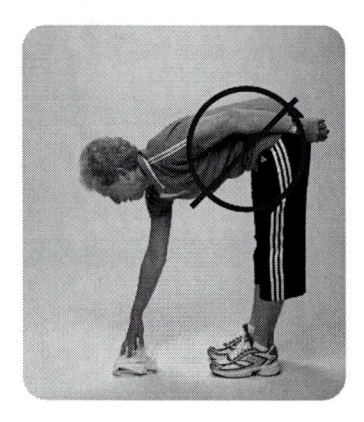

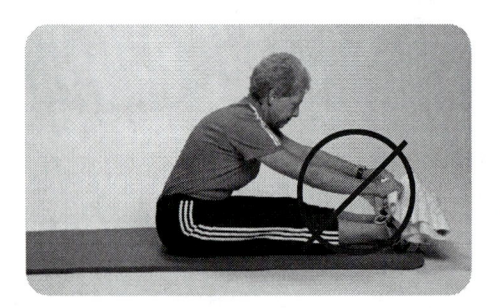

Don't let the affected leg cross midline of the body.

- Don't cross the legs while sitting or sleeping.

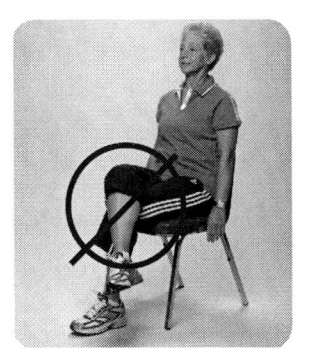

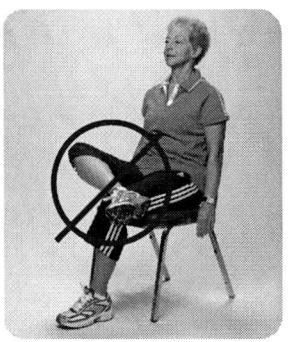

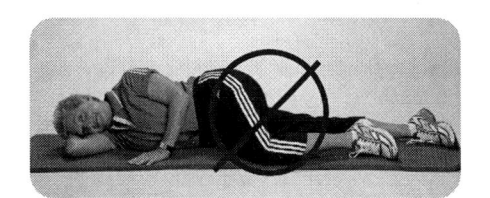

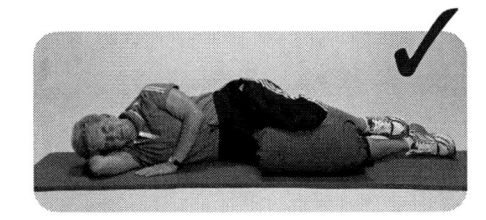

- Place a pillow between the legs to maintain alignment.

Don't rotate the leg too far inward or outward when standing, walking, or turning.

- Don't stand pigeon-toed.
- Don't plant the foot and turn the body.

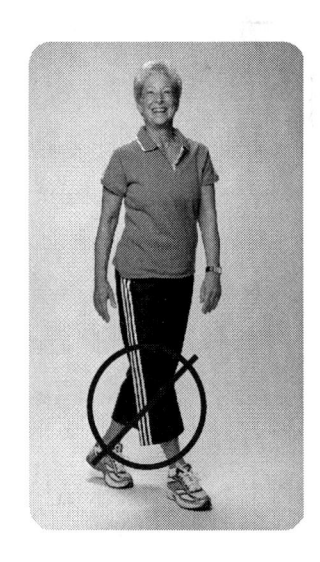

Study Questions

Complete the following questions. The answer key is on pages 85–86.

1. Name the three risk factors that negatively affect joint replacement postoperative outcomes.

    (1) *Obesity*

    (2) *Diabtes*

    (3) *Hypertension*

2. List three hip precautions a client must follow to avoid dislocating a hip replacement.

    (1) *not bend beyond 90° angle*

    (2) *don't cross leg*

    (3) *don't rotate leg in/out*

3. List three safe activities and three high-risk activities for a client with total joint replacement to participate in.

safe	not safe
    (1) *walking* / *jogging*
    (2) *swimming* / *skiing*
    (3) *golfing* / *Tennis*

4. True or false. Complications of a total joint replacement include dislocation, infection, and loosening. *(True circled)*

CHAPTER 3

Health Screening and Client Assessment

This section outlines your responsibilities as a professional fitness practitioner. It is not meant to be comprehensive but is a reminder of the responsibilities of a health fitness professional working with clients who have had total joint replacements. Professional responsibilities include information on health screening, medical clearance, fitness assessment, monitoring exercise, record keeping, emergency procedures, scope of practice, and physician referral.

Health Screening for Physical Activity

Health screening is a crucial first step in maintaining the safety and effectiveness of any exercise program. Health screening has several purposes, including identifying health conditions and risk factors that put your client at risk when participating in an exercise program or may necessitate referral to a healthcare professional; assisting in the design of an appropriate exercise program; identifying possible contraindicated activities; fulfilling legal and insurance requirements for you or your facility; and encouraging and maintaining communication with the client's healthcare provider.

The Physical Activity Readiness Questionnaire (PAR-Q) has been recommended as a minimal standard for entry into low- to moderate-intensity exercise programs (ACSM, 2006; AACVPR, 2004). More detailed medical/health history forms may be appropriate for clients with chronic disease or disabilities. A health-screening process is a valuable tool that will assist the fitness practitioner in safely and appropriately individualizing the client's exercise program. Information on the form should be referred to often and updated every year or when a new condition arises.

Previous Exercise Level and Restrictions

The client assessment should include a history of the client's rehabilitation experience either in an inpatient facility or outpatient setting. This will give the fitness professional an idea of what type of training the client has performed and which exercises he or she might already be familiar with. Some clients will have continued to perform an exercise program designed for them by a physical therapist. Ask the client when he or she last saw the orthopedic surgeon who performed the surgery. It is important to inquire whether the client has been given any specific restrictions from the doctor. Sometimes the client is not to lift anything over 40 pounds since this places added stress through the lower extremity and places the patient in unsafe postures. Some clients must follow the hip precautions if they have had a total hip replacement performed. If you have any doubts about the appropriate activity level or restrictions for the client, do not hesitate to contact the physician or the physical therapist for guidance.

In addition to the general medical health-screening form, the following questions specific to the client's joint replacement surgery are helpful in designing a safe and effective exercise program.

- When was your surgery?
- What specific type of surgery did you undergo?
- Is your prosthesis cemented or noncemented?
- What type of rehabilitation did you have after being discharged from the hospital?
- When was your last visit to the orthopedic surgeon?

- When was the last time you worked with a physical therapist and where was it? (at the hospital, at home, or as an outpatient)
- What is your correct weight-bearing status?
- If you are fully weight bearing, how long have you been allowed to put full weight on the leg?
- Have you been performing any type of exercise at home?
- Has the physician given you any specific restrictions?
- Are you still observing the hip precautions?
- Do you know what the hip precautions are?

Remember that the health-screening process should always be followed by careful monitoring and observation during the exercise session.

Medical Clearance

If indicated by the PAR-Q or the health-screening instrument, the client should be referred to his or her healthcare provider for medical clearance. It is strongly advised that clients with special medical conditions, identified as "at risk" or exhibiting symptoms during an exercise bout, obtain a medical clearance from his or her physician prior to the start of any exercise program. The American College of Sports Medicine (ACSM) has recommended criteria for situations that warrant a physician's release prior to exercise.

Fitness professionals reserve the right to require any participant, upon reviewing his or her medical history form, to provide a physician's release prior to the admittance to an exercise program and reserve the right to screen individuals from a program who are deemed medically inappropriate. It is important that any physician-signed release that contains specific recommendations, modifications, or restrictions be fully respected and adhered to by the fitness practitioner. Always clarify the upper safe limit of exercise and other restrictions with clients and their physician.

Medications

The health history form should identify any prescription or over-the-counter medications your client is taking. Some medications will influence the heart's response to exercise and your client's exercise tolerance. Other medications, such as pain relievers, dull pain symptoms that may occur during the exercise program. Therefore, be aware of any complaints of pain from the client and modify the exercises appropriately. The *Physician's Desk Reference* (PDR) is an excellent reference text for seeking more detailed information regarding prescription medications. If you have any questions regarding the client's health history, medical status, medication, or physician's release, contact the physician directly.

Monitoring Exercise

Several effective methods can be used to monitor exercise. Minimum routine monitoring should include heart rate and perceived exertion. In clients with known cardiovascular disease, blood pressure should be monitored.

Heart Rate

The trainer should encourage clients to learn to palpate and count their own heart rate (HR), if possible. However, some clients have lost sensation in the finger pads and may be unable to perform this task. If a client has difficulty finding the pulse at the radial artery, try the caratid artery.

Perceived Exertion

The BORG Rating of Perceived Exertion (RPE scale) is an acceptable way to monitor exercise intensity and tolerance. This method works well when used in conjunction with HR monitoring. This is the preferred method for older clients or for those on HR-lowering medication, with pain-limiting symptoms, or those unable to palpate their pulse rate. Perceived exertion is also recommended for clients with exertional angina, claudication, or who are extremely deconditioned. The RPE should be compatible with the client's physical appearance and response to the exercise.

Numerical Pain Scale

A numerical pain rating scale can be used to rate the client's pain or discomfort during or after exercise. A 0 on the scale is equivalent to no pain, and 10 means the pain is the worst possible. Moderate pain would be around the middle of the scale, or rated close to 5, while 2 or 3 would be mild pain. The number 7 or higher is equal to severe pain and indicates that some type of exercise routine modification is necessary. If pain greater than 7 persists, have the client call or return to see the physician as soon as possible. If the pain is around 2 or 3, ask the client if any specific exercises are uncomfortable and remove them from the routine until the pain subsides. When in doubt, always contact the physician!

Physical Observation

Practitioners, as well as clients, should be taught to observe physical signs or symptoms that indicate overwork. Signals of overwork include abnormal musculoskeletal pain or discomfort, an elevated heart rate that is above what is normal for the client, red face, abnormal shortness of breath with exercise, excessive perspiration, abnormal fatigue, chest pains or palpitations, and excessive fatigue or discomfort. In addition, clients should be instructed not to exercise during an acute illness, when fatigued, or under excessive stress. Clients should be taught to identify inappropriate responses to exercise and to report their occurrence.

Re-Entry to Exercise

Clients returning to exercise may require several days to several weeks to regain their original exercise workloads. They should begin activity at a lesser intensity and gradually progress to higher exercise levels. Re-entry at too rapid a pace can cause increased pain and undesirable stress to the joint.

Record Keeping

Record keeping is an integral part of any exercise program and is important to demonstrate objective improvement to the client, practitioner, and healthcare provider and to assist in guiding the progression of exercise. It is helpful in determining normal and abnormal responses to exercise training. This is particularly true for heart rate and blood pressure responses at rest and exercise, as well as musculoskeletal pain or fatigue that may occur during or after exercise. If the client were to have any problem during or after the exercise, documentation of exercise progression and tolerance would be important. Any changes in medication or physician recommendations should be noted and adhered to.

Be sure to note any abnormal responses to exercise that may occur during a session. This information can be recorded on the client's daily workout log for the individual training day. It should be noted that clients whose function is not maintained or who do not improve with adequate adherence to appropriate exercise may require physician evaluation.

Establishing Physician Contact

Establishing and developing contact and rapport with the medical community will greatly enhance your ability to provide for your clients with joint replacements. There are benefits in developing relationships between the physician and fitness practitioner for the client, as well as the involved professionals. First, it ensures a safe program for clients and establishes credibility with physicians and healthcare providers. Second, it builds a potential referral system between the fitness practitioner and the medical community. It also is an excellent way to obtain educational information for the fitness trainer, as well as for the physician.

Scope of Practice

It is vitally important for your client's safety and your own to work within the limit and scope of your professional training and qualifications. Performing therapeutic treatments, recommending dietary changes or nutritional supplements for the treatment of joint disease, or modifying a client's prescribed medication dosage are just a few of the tasks that are beyond an exercise practitioner's scope of practice. Do not try to diagnose a joint replacement complication if you notice possible signs or symptoms. Instead, inform the patient that it is very important for them to see the physician promptly. Finally, assume the client needs to follow hip precautions while exercising, unless otherwise informed by the client, physical therapist, or the physician.

Physician Referral

Inappropriate responses to exercise that are persistent, that indicate termination of exercise, or that occur consistently should be referred to the client's physician or healthcare provider. Reasons to refer your joint-replacement client to his or her physician include (1) increased pain in the surgical region or consistent pain that does not decrease over time; (2) pain, swelling, warmth, or redness in the calf; and (3) decrease in overall health condition or new health complaints. If there is ever any doubt of the appropriateness of exercise, check with your medical advisor or the client's physician.

Emergency Procedures

It is important to know emergency medical procedures and have a system in place for responding to a medical emergency. An emergency plan must be devised for every training situation. In a medical emergency, the person needs medical help immediately. Act quickly and insist on prompt medical attention, even if the person resists.

First, call an emergency rescue service by dialing "911" on a phone. While waiting for emergency medical services to arrive, keep the person quiet, in a half-sitting position, and try to relieve his/her anxiety. Loosen tight-fitting clothing and maintain an even body temperature. Do not lift the person or give him/her food or drink. If the person is unconscious:

- Check his/her breathing. If the person is not breathing and if you are qualified to do so, initiate artificial respiration.
- Check for the heartbeat. If the person is not breathing and there is no pulse, initiate CPR until medical help arrives, but only if you are trained to perform CPR.

- If your worksite has an AED (automated external defibrillator) and you have been trained in its use, then use it.

Emergency treatment aims to restore normal heartbeat and blood flow as quickly as possible. Once the person is in the hands of a trained medical professional, medications will be administered to stabilize heart rate, BP, and to relieve pain.

Other medications that may be administered to the person are:

- Pain relievers
- Medications that control blood pressure and heart rhythms
- Medications to relax the patient and reduce the stress of the event
- Oxygen
- Defibrillation or electric shock, which may be necessary to restore or correct the heartbeat.

Throughout the medical treatment process there is continuous monitoring of all vital signs.

Client Assessment

Assessing the joint-replacement client is important for two reasons: (1) to have a baseline from which to measure the client's progress, and (2) to develop a safe and effective exercise program that will improve the client's gait pattern, range of motion, strength, and balance.

Gait Pattern

After undergoing a total joint replacement in the lower extremity, a client may have some form of ambulation abnormality. An ambulation abnormality can be due to muscle weakness, continued pain in the limb, or a developed habit. Some clients will not have any visible deficits, but muscular testing will indicate weakness in the areas associated with the joint-replacement surgery. This is particularly true of the gluteus medius following hip replacement surgery. Two of the most common gait pattern abnormalities are discussed below.

Antalgic Gait Pattern

An antalgic gait pattern is one in which the person limps, usually due to pain. The person does not put full weight on the limb and quickly transfers the weight off the involved leg. Clients who present with an antalgic gait pattern may want to achieve ambulating without a limp or walking without an assistive device such as a cane.

Trendelenburg Gait Pattern

The Trendelenburg gait pattern is mostly associated with total hip replacement. This pattern is a result of weakness of the gluteus medius. The gluteus medius is responsible for stabilizing the hip while walking. If the gluteus medius muscle is weak, you will see the opposite hip dip down when standing on the weak hip. For example, a client who has had a right hip replacement and the right hip is still very weak. If that client has a Trendelenburg gait pattern when walking, you will see the client's left hip dip down when weight is transferred to the right side.

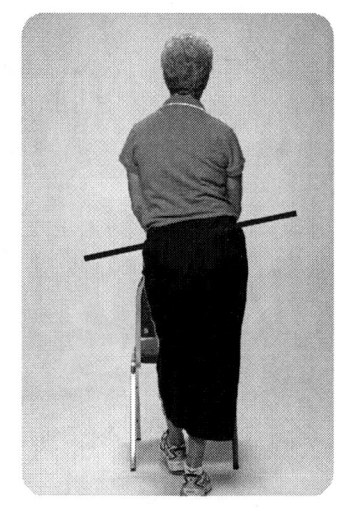

Right hip weakness.

Although a physician or physical therapist would formally assess and document this condition, a personal trainer with keen observation skills can see this type of gait pattern. With specific strengthening of the gluteus medius, this ambulation abnormality will diminish.

Range of Motion

Adequate range of motion of the hip and knee joints is needed to perform a variety of functional activities, such as getting in and out of a chair or bath tub, climbing stairs, and walking properly. Knee joint range of motion after a total knee replacement is critical to the ultimate success of the client returning to a normal activity level.

Knee Joint Range of Motion

Normal knee joint extension measures approximately 0 degrees, meaning the knee is fully straightened. Knee flexion for the normal client should be around 130 degrees. Evaluating the range of motion for a total knee replacement client will give you an idea of which muscles require flexibility training. If the knee is 30 degrees away from being straight, it would be important to stretch the hamstring muscle as part of the client's program. Likewise, if the knee only bends to 90 degrees, the flexibility of the quadriceps should be increased. Recording the approximate joint range of motion during the assessment will help track the client's progress throughout the workout sessions.

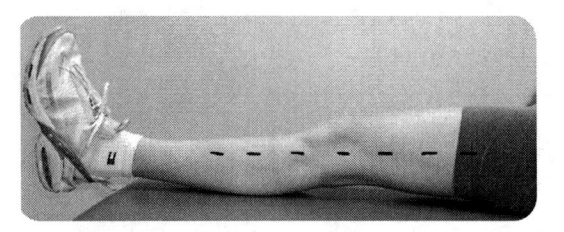

Normal knee extension (0 degrees)

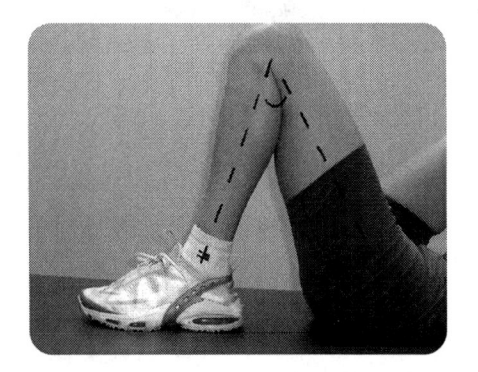

Normal knee flexion (130 degrees)

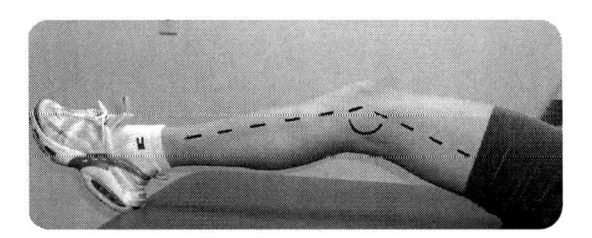

Knee flexion 30 degrees

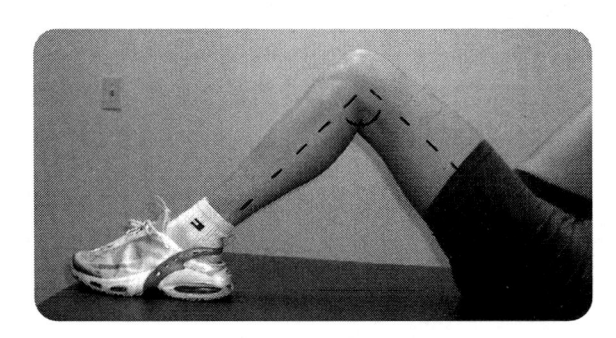

Knee flexion 90 degrees

Hip Joint Range of Motion

It is not necessary to measure the hip range of motion in a client who has had a total hip replacement. Placing clients in certain positions to look at hip range of motion may place them at risk for hip dislocation. As long as the client is able to sit normally, the hip joint range of motion should be within normal limits. Tight hip flexors may need to be addressed in some clients.

Muscle Strength

Strength is a very important aspect of fitness training and especially important after a total joint replacement. The knee and hip joints are the two main weight-bearing joints in the body. Without proper strength a person cannot walk, transfer in and out of chair, or balance properly. The following tests give the fitness professional an idea of the client's strength in the lower extremity musculature.

Quadriceps

A gross assessment of quadriceps strength can be made by having the client sit on the edge of a table or bench. Place one hand over the ankle and stabilize the thigh with your other hand. Have the client attempt to straighten the leg against the resistance. A client who lacks full quadriceps strength may not be able to push strongly enough to move the resisting hand away.

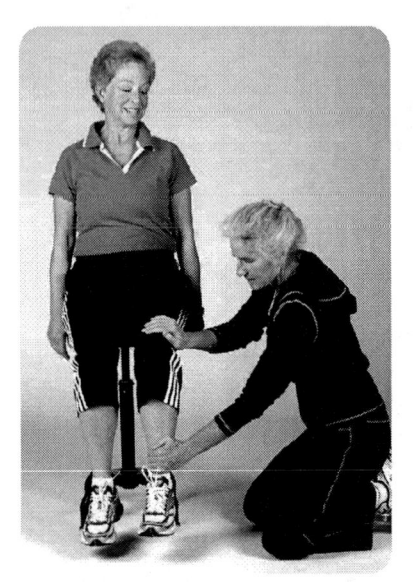

Assessing quadriceps strength

Hamstrings

To test the strength of the hamstrings, position the client sitting over the edge of a table or bench. Place one hand behind the client's lower leg and stabilize the thigh with your other hand. The client begins the test with the leg slightly extended and then attempts to bend the knee against the resistance. A client who lacks full hamstring strength may not be able to pull strongly enough to move the resisting hand toward the table.

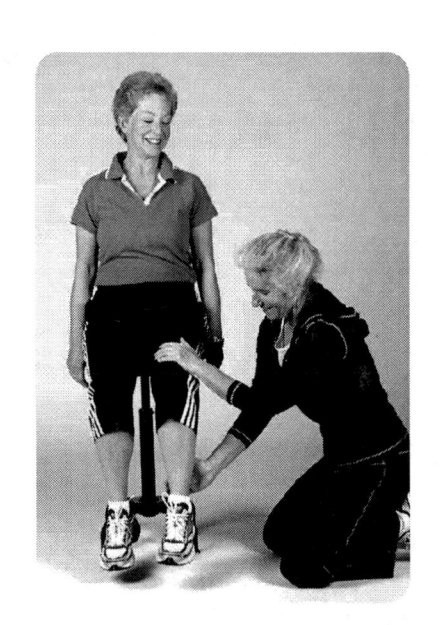

Assessing hamstrings strength

Gluteus Maximus

Position the client standing on one leg holding onto a chair, wall, or table for support with the leg to be tested lifted off the ground. Place one hand on the back of the thigh and place the other hand over the foot. The client should then attempt to extend the hip against the resistance of the hand on the thigh. The knee should be kept bent throughout the test to minimize the substitution of the hamstrings. A client who lacks full gluteus maximus strength may not be able to lift the hip or push against the manual resistance.

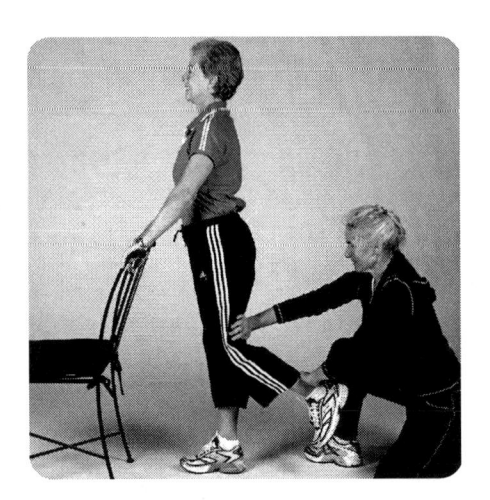

Assessing gluteus maximus strength

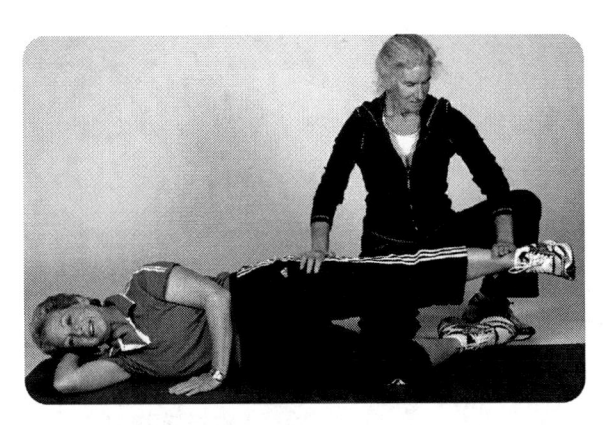

Gluteus Medius

To test this muscle the client lies with the side to be tested up toward the ceiling. The bottom knee is bent and the upper leg is straight and in slight hip external rotation. The pelvis should be stabilized with one hand. Ask the client to lift the leg. Apply light resistance at the ankle if the client is able to lift the leg easily. Weakness of the gluteus medius is observed when the client is unable to hold the leg up, begins to have cramping, or attempts to rotate the pelvis backward to employ other muscles.

Assessing gluteus medius strength

Single-Leg Stance

By asking the client to stand on one foot and hold that position, you can test both balance and overall muscle strength of the supporting leg. This test is appropriate for both total knee and total hip replacement clients. Some clients who have had a total hip replacement may be unable to keep their hips level. To determine if the client's gluteus medius muscle is weak, have the client stand on the surgical leg and note whether the opposite hip dips down. The gluteus medius muscle keeps the hips level. If the opposite hip drops, it indicates weakness of the gluteus medius muscle on the standing leg.

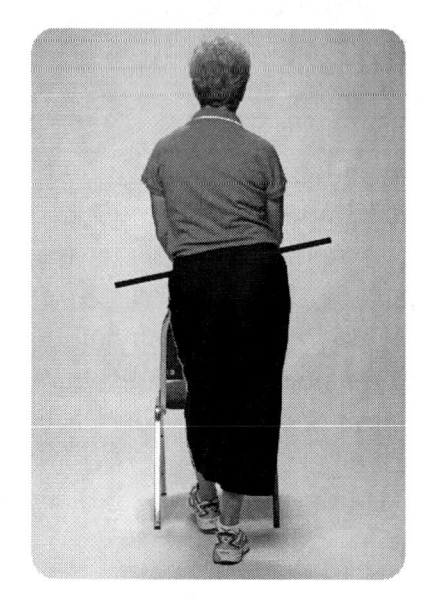

Muscle Girth

A 2005 study on total knee replacement patients (Mizner, et al.) not only showed a 62% decrease in quadriceps strength, but also found a 10% decrease in maximal cross-sectional quadriceps area compared with preoperative measurements. Muscle atrophy can be subtle, so taking an objective measurement may help to quantify this loss of muscle girth. This measurement is most appropriate for total knee replacement clients.

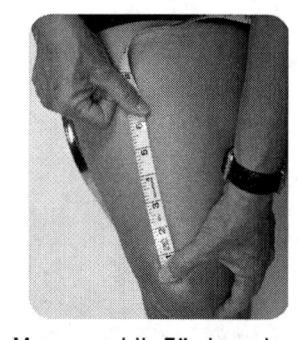

Measure girth 5" above knee

To measure muscle girth of the quadriceps, wrap a tape measure around the thigh approximately 5 inches above the knee joint line. Measure both thighs for comparison. Be aware that swelling around the knee can interfere with a true reading of the muscle girth.

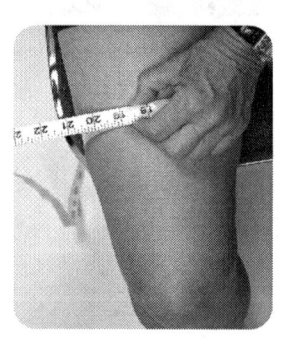

Girth measurement

Fitness Evaluations

Fitness evaluations are an integral part of the health-screening process. They are used to assess parameters of fitness, assign beginning workloads, and serve as a baseline for future comparisons. Standard resting assessments include height, weight, resting heart rate, and resting blood pressure. Standard field tests for flexibility, muscle strength, muscle endurance, sub-maximal cardiovascular endurance, and body composition may be administered. Established field assessments are easily administered and are reliable methods to determine initial fitness levels, client's exercise tolerance, limiting symptoms, and to monitor changes in fitness resulting from the exercise program.

Keep in mind, standard field tests may not always be appropriate for clients with total joint replacements due to symptom limitations and hip precautions following hip replacement surgery. Professional judgment and weighing the benefits and the risks, both physical and psychological, should be used before blindly administering fitness assessments. During any assessment, it is important to have the client note any unusual pain, fatigue, or symptomology that may be present.

Study Questions

Complete the following questions. The answer key is on page 86.

1. True or false. A Trendelenburg gait pattern occurs when the gluteus maximus is weak on the side of the operation.

2. True or false. Normal knee range of motion is approximately 10 degrees of extension to 140 degrees of flexion.

3. List five specific health screening questions for the client who has had knee or hip joint replacement surgery.

    (1) _____

    (2) _____

    (3) _____

    (4) _____

    (5) _____

4. Name three appropriate ways to monitor exercise.

    (1) _____

    (2) _____

    (3) _____

5. True or false. The strength of the quadriceps is tested by asking the client to bend the knee against the resistance of the personal trainer's hand.

6. Name the test that evaluates the overall muscle strength of the supporting leg, as well as the client's balance.

    _____

CHAPTER 4

Exercises

The exercises in this chapter are presented in the following format: Exercises for each joint are organized into beginner, intermediate, and advanced. The primary muscles that are used in each exercise are listed, the positioning and execution of the exercises are described, and any client reminders or common mistakes are provided. Finally, modifications are provided to progress the client as needed. All exercise should be performed in a slow and controlled manner.

Total Knee Replacement Exercises

The most important muscles to strengthen after a total knee replacement are the muscles that surround the joint, specifically the quadriceps muscle. The hamstring muscles as they cross the knee joint can be inflexible from being in a protective position after surgery due to postsurgical pain. For this reason it is important to emphasize quadriceps strengthening and hamstring flexibility. Stretching the hamstrings is important throughout the training process and may be performed at home between formal training sessions.

Beginner Exercises

These exercises can be used for clients who are deconditioned, have not exercised in awhile, or who still have limitations in their knee strength and range of motion. As previously mentioned, the full range of motion for the knee joint is

48   Chapter 4

0 degrees to 130 degrees. Many clients will not regain this full range of motion, but should work toward regaining as much knee extension and flexion as possible. The following are open-kinetic-chain exercises that emphasize overall strength. Open-kinetic-chain exercises place less pressure on the limb and joints because they are performed without putting weight on the floor.

Quadriceps Push   quadriceps

The quadriceps muscle group is made up of the rectus femoris, vastus lateralis, vastus intermedius, and vastus medialis.

Positioning Sit on a mat or lie on the back with the involved leg straight.

Execution Push the back of the knee down toward the mat, attempting to straighten the leg as much as possible. Hold for 5 seconds.

Client reminder Tighten the muscle on the front of the thigh.

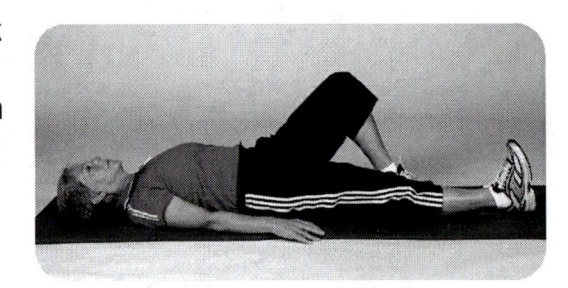

Common error Using the buttocks instead of the quadriceps to push the leg down.

Modification A small rolled towel can be placed underneath the knee if the leg is uncomfortable in the straightened position.

Straight Leg Lift   quadriceps and iliopsoas

Positioning Lie flat or propped on the elbows with the involved leg straight. Bend the opposite knee.

Execution Keeping the knee straight, lift the leg approximately 12 inches off the mat. Hold for 5 seconds.

Client reminder Keep the leg straight.

Common error Allowing the knee to bend and lifting primarily with the hip flexors.

Modification Add weights close to the knee at first then place them closer to the ankle to make the exercise more challenging.

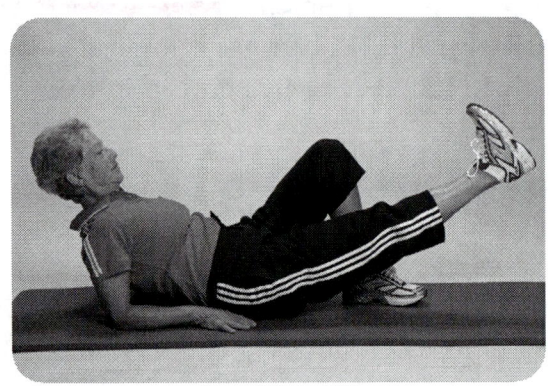

Straight Leg Lift with Toe Out **quadriceps, especially the vastus medialis and iliopsoas**

Positioning Lie flat or propped on the elbows. With the opposite leg bent, straighten the involved leg and turn the toe outward.

Execution Keeping the knee straight, lift the leg approximately 12 inches off the mat. Hold for 5 seconds.

Client reminder Keep the leg straight.

Common error Allowing the knee to bend and lifting primarily with the hip flexors.

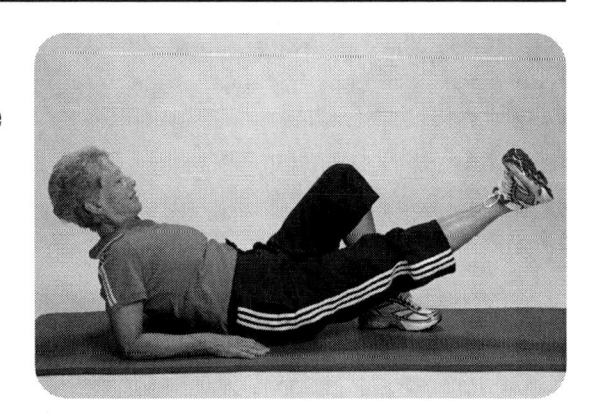

Modification Add weights close to the knee at first then place them closer to the ankle to make the exercise more challenging.

Leg Kick-Out **quadriceps**

Positioning Sit on a table, bench, or chair.

Execution Straighten the knee fully and hold for 5 seconds.

Client reminder Keep the thigh supported.

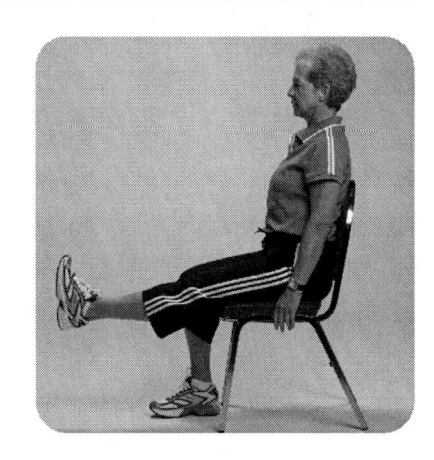

Modification Add weights close to the knee at first then place them closer to the ankle to make the exercise more challenging.

Sidelying Abduction   quadriceps, especially the vastus lateralis, gluteus medius, and gluteus minimus strength

Positioning Lie on the side opposite of the involved joint. Bend the knee on the bottom and keep the upper knee straight.

Execution Lift the straight leg off the bottom leg. Hold for 5 seconds.

Client reminders Keep the leg straight. Do not let the hips drop forward or backward.

Modification Add weights close to the knee at first then place them closer to the ankle to make the exercise more challenging.

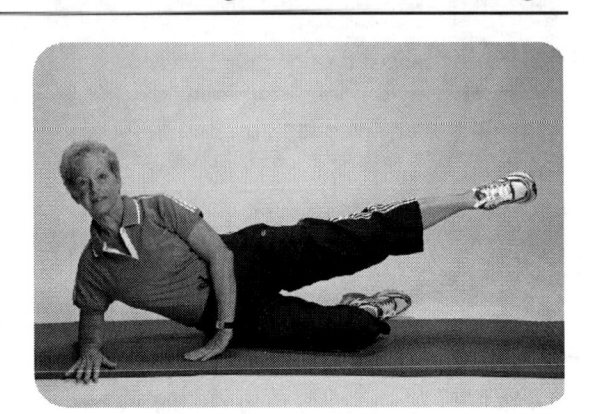

Sidelying Adduction   adductor group and quadriceps, especially the vastus medialis

The adductor muscle group consists of the adductor magnus, adductor longus, and adductor brevis.

Positioning Lie on the side of the involved joint. Place the sole of the top foot behind the straightened bottom leg.

Execution Lift the bottom leg up off the mat. Hold for 5 seconds.

Client reminders Keep the leg straight. Do not let the hips drop forward or backward.

Modifications Use a stool and place the upper leg on top of it. Lift the involved leg to the underside of the stool. Add weights close to the knee at first then place them closer to the ankle to make the exercise more challenging.

Flexibility Exercises

Increasing and maintaining flexibility is crucial following a total knee replacement. Many clients will have had extensive physical therapy to ensure their range of motion was adequate to perform functional activities such as getting up from a chair and climbing stairs. These flexibility exercises should be incorporated into the client's workout whether or not they have residual limitations in their range of motion.

Supine Hamstrings Stretch   medial and lateral hamstring flexibility

The medial hamstrings consist of the semitendinosis and the semimembranosus. The lateral hamstring is the biceps femoris.

Positioning Lie on the back.

Execution Lift the leg toward the ceiling and hold on to the back of the thigh. Hold for 20–30 seconds. Repeat 3–5 times.

Client reminder Keep the knee as straight as possible.

Modification Place a towel or strap around the arch of the foot to assist the stretch.

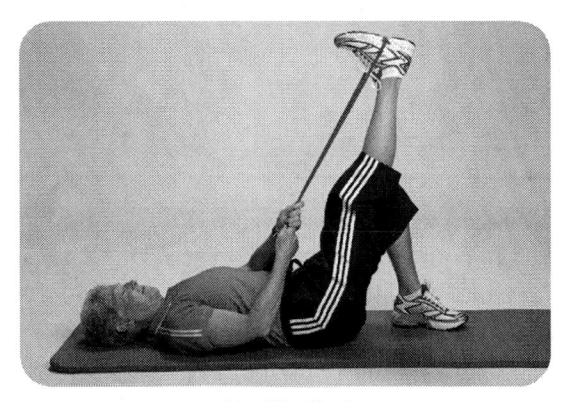

(Modification)

Standing Hamstrings Stretch   medial and lateral hamstrings

Positioning Standing, prop one heel on a stool or step.

Execution Lean forward at the waist with the trunk straight. Hold 20–30 seconds. Repeat 3–5 times.

Client reminder Keep the back flat and the knee straight.

Common errors Rounding the back. Putting the foot flat on the stool.

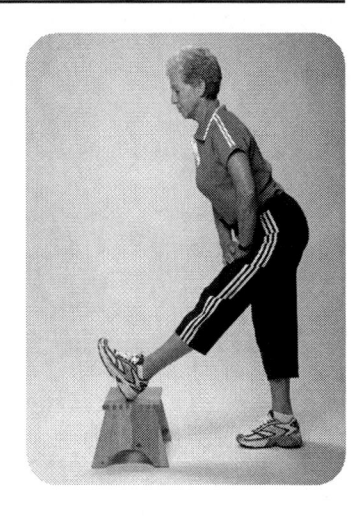

Heel to Buttocks

quadriceps

Positioning Lie prone on a mat.

Execution With towel or strap wrapped around the foot or ankle of the involved leg, bend the knee and pull the foot toward the buttocks. Hold for 20–30 seconds. Repeat 3–5 times.

Common error Twisting away from the side that is being stretched.

Modification If the client is sensitive to pressure on the anterior thigh, place a towel underneath the distal thigh of the leg being stretched.

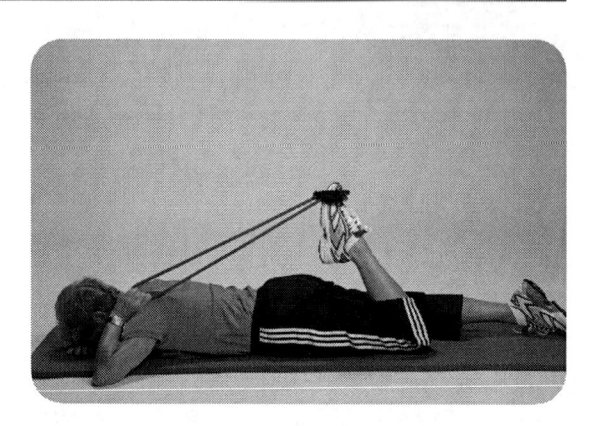

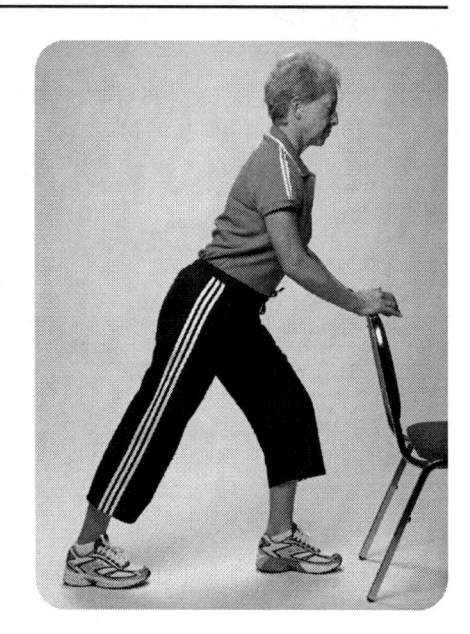

Calf Stretch

gastrocnemius

Positioning Standing, place both hands against a wall or chair for support and place one foot behind the other.

Execution Bend the front knee toward the wall and keep the back knee straight. Hold for 20–30 seconds. Repeat 3–5 times.

Client reminder Press the back heel into the floor.

Common error Feet too far apart. Allowing the back heel to lift off the floor.

Calf Stretch on Step   **gastrocnemius**

Positioning Stand on a stool or step. A support can be used for balance. Bring one heel off the edge of the step.

Execution Drop the heel below the step, keeping the knee straight. Slightly bend the knee that is standing on step. Hold for 20–30 seconds. Repeat 3–5 times.

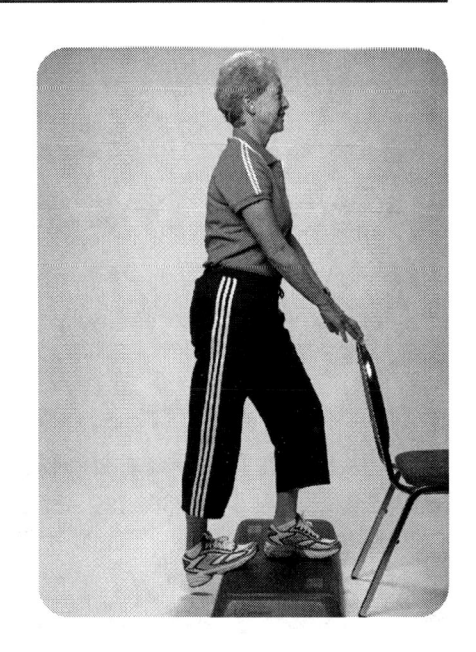

Cardiovascular Endurance

Use any of the following machines for 10 to 25 minutes to improve endurance, strength, and flexibility. Cardiovascular conditioning can be used throughout the training process.

Recumbent Bicycle

Positioning Each knee should have a slight bend when the leg is at the most extended position.

Treadmill

Begin without an incline. The treadmill can also be used to reinforce proper gait pattern with slow walking.

Elliptical Machine

The elliptical machine gives a full-body workout and requires greater knee range of motion to perform this more advanced exercise properly.

Intermediate Exercises

These exercises are for clients who have good knee range of motion and are working to improve their lower body strength.

Standing Knee Extension   quadriceps

Positioning Stand with the resisted band around the upper portion of the calf with the other portion of the band attached to something sturdy. Begin with the knee slightly bent.
Execution Straighten the knee against the resistance of the band.
Client reminders Perform exercises in a slow and controlled manner.
Common error Pulling back with the hip and not the knee.
Modification Increase the resistance of the band.

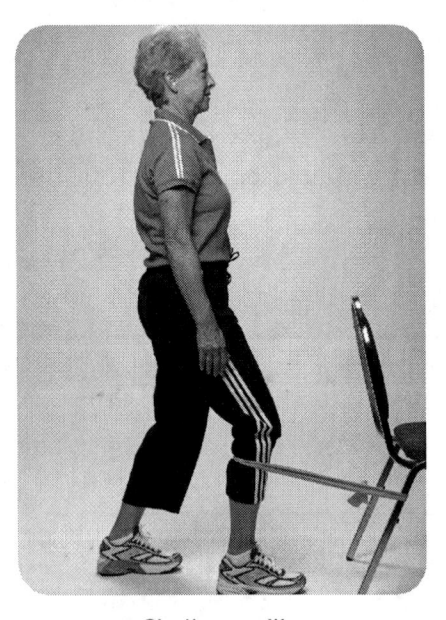

Starting position

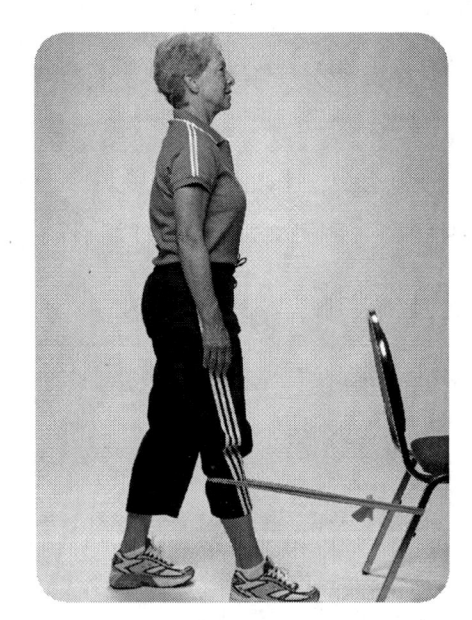

Ending position

Resisted-Band Leg Pulls

Positioning Stand with the resisted band around the ankle and the other portion of the band attached to something sturdy. Use a support for balance if needed.

Execution This exercise can be performed in four different directions: hip flexion, hip extension, hip abduction, and hip adduction.

Client reminders Perform exercises in a slow and controlled manner. Stand up straight and do not lean forward or to the side. Keep knee of active leg straight but not locked.

Common errors Bending the knee of the active leg. Leaning forward while pulling band back.

Modification Increase the resistance of the band.

Note The client will often feel a greater strain on the leg they are standing on than the leg they are pulling the band with. The progression should be: (1) involved leg pulling the band and (2) standing on the involved leg and pulling the band with the other leg.

Flexion   quadriceps and iliopsoas

Execution Pull band forward, keeping the knee straight.

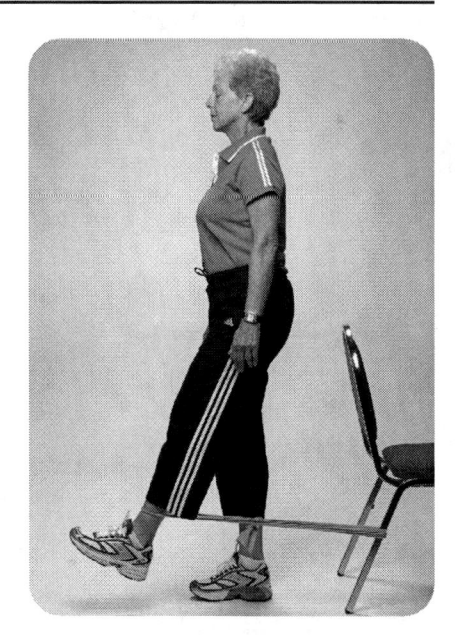

Extension   quadriceps, gluteus maximus, and hamstrings

Execution Pull band backward, keeping the knee straight.

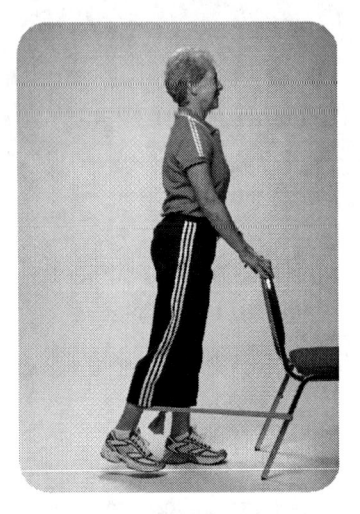

Abduction   quadriceps, especially the vastus lateralis, gluteus medius, and minimus

Execution Pull band out to the side, keeping the knee straight.

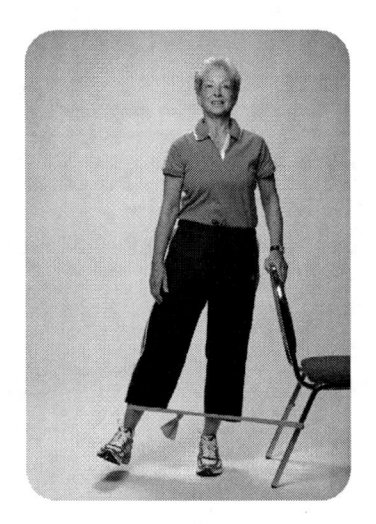

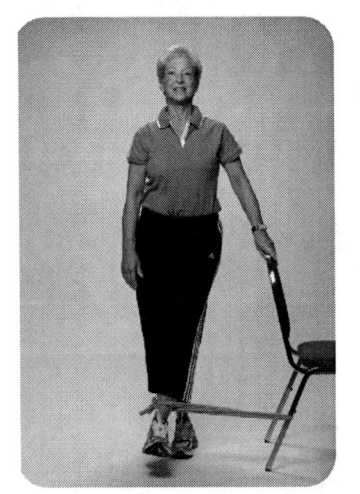

Adduction   quadriceps, especially the vastus medialis, adductor group, and gracilis

Execution Pull band in toward midline, keeping knee straight.

Wall Squats

quadriceps and gluteals

Positioning Rest the back on the wall with both feet approximately 2–3 feet from the wall. Make sure the knees are not farther out than the toes.

Execution Slide the back down the wall and hold for 5 seconds. Straighten both knees and slide back to starting position.

Client reminder Do not let the knees go over toes.

Modifications Use an inflatable ball behind the small of the back when sliding down the wall. Sit and hold the squat for 10–30 seconds.

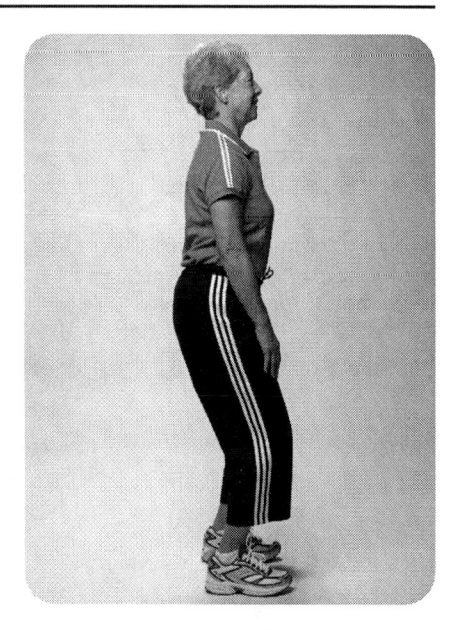

Resisted-Band Squats

quadriceps and gluteals

Positioning Stand on a resisted band with feet shoulder-width apart. Hold on to the ends of the band.

Execution Bend knees while holding the band in the same position. Straighten knees slowly against the resistance of the band. Keep back flat.

Common error Losing tension in the band during the exercise and too much knee flexion and not enough hip flexion.

Modification Increase resistance of the band.

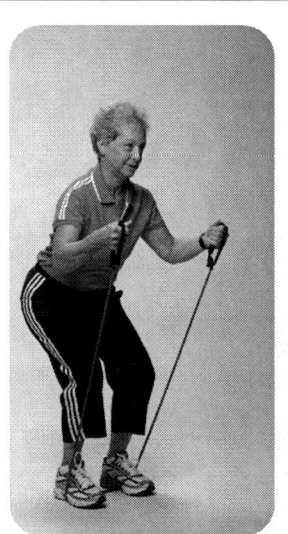

Start position   End position

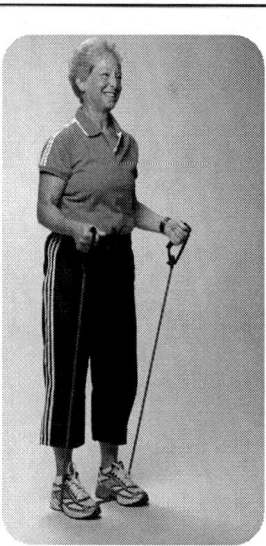

Steps*

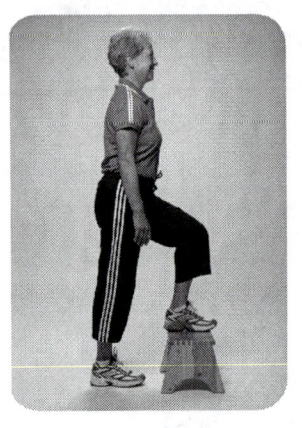

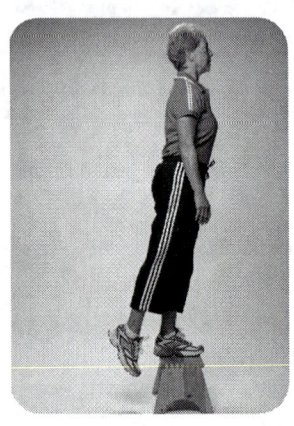

Forward **quadriceps**

Execution Facing the stool, step up with the involved leg.

Backward
quadriceps, gluteals, and hamstrings

Execution Standing on the stool, step down to the floor, keeping the involved leg on the stool. Step back up onto the stool.

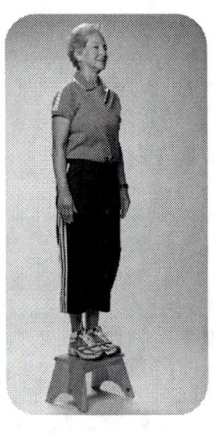

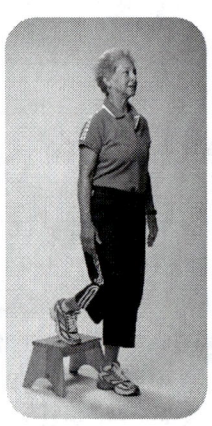

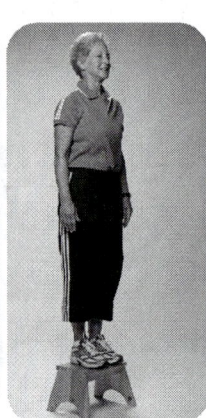

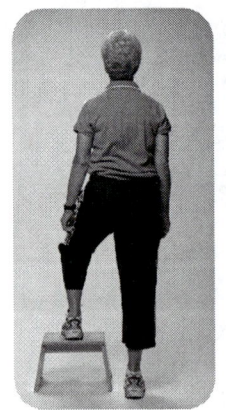

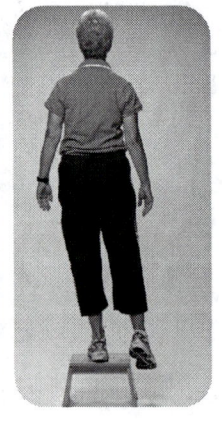

Lateral
quadriceps, especially the vastus lateralis, gluteus medius, and minimus

Execution Standing with the stool next to the involved leg and step sideways onto the stool.

*A support can be used to hold onto for balance if needed when performing step exercises.

Advanced Exercises

These exercises are for clients who have had physical therapy in the past and/or have been exercising regularly after their operation. The machine exercises are placed in the advanced section because they can be progressed to a much higher resistance than the other exercises.

The resistance while performing the band exercises is different from the resistance of the machines. The bands have greater resistance the farther they are stretched. The machines are a form of isotonic exercise, which keeps the amount of weight the same throughout the range of motion. Although the machines have a greater overall resistance capacity, it may be more appropriate to use the bands depending on the client's goals. In addition, the bands can easily be used at home. All of the machine exercises can be made more challenging by adding weight in a progressive manner.

Hip Resistance Machine — hip flexor, extensor, abductor, and adductor muscle groups, knee flexor and extensor groups

Although this machine emphasizes hip motion, knee strength is required to stabilize on the stationary or standing leg. For example, if the client has had a left total knee replacement, he or she may be more challenged by standing on the left leg while performing the exercises with the right leg.

Because each machine is slightly different, a full explanation of the execution of the exercise will not be given. Keep in mind that the exercises can be performed in four different directions of the hip, including flexion, extension, abduction, and adduction.

Leg Press — quadriceps and gluteus maximus

Positioning Lie facing up on the "sled" with feet on the foot plate.
Execution Push the sled away as the feet remain stationary.
Modification The reverse motion is possible with other types of machines where the plate is pushed away and the body remains stationary.
Client reminder The knees should not move forward of the toes.

Knee Extension Machine   quadriceps

Positioning Seated with the bar over the shins.

Execution Straighten knees without locking them.

Note This exercise should **not** be performed with the involved leg only because it places a great deal of torque through the knee joint.

Hamstring Curl Machine   hamstrings and gluteus maximus

Positioning Lie prone on the machine with the bar above the ankle line.

Execution Bend knees and pull bar toward buttocks.

Note If the involved knee is lacking a great deal of knee extension range of motion, it is not appropriate to perform this exercise. It is essential for the client to have adequate hamstring flexibility before focusing on knee flexion or hamstring strength.

Sideways Walking with Elastic Band   quadriceps and gluteals

Positioning Place a resisted band, tied in a knot, around the lower legs.

Execution Step sideways with the band kept tight and the knees partially bent. Repeat for 10–20 feet.

Client reminder Use the outside of the thighs and take large steps.

Modification Increase resistance of the band or increase the depth of the squat.

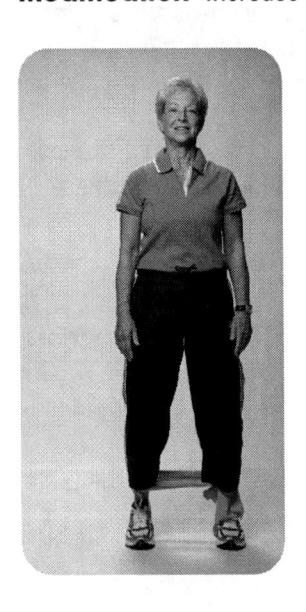

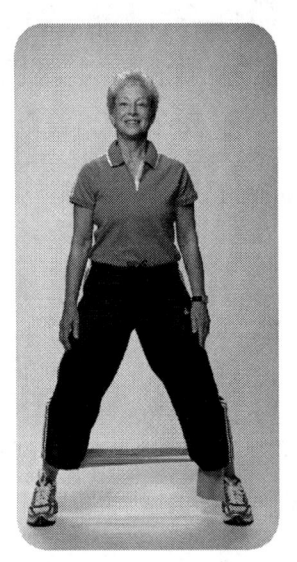

Step Taps   requires good eccentric muscle control of the quadriceps, hip stability strength, and gastrocnemius flexibility

Positioning Stand on a stool or small step. These exercises should be performed holding onto a support for balance.

Execution While standing on the involved leg, squat slightly until the toe of the opposite leg is touching the ground. Immediately straighten the leg on the step so weight is not placed on the foot tapping the ground.

Client reminders Bend the support knee to place the toe on the floor. Avoid reaching with the toe.

Modification Increase the height of the step to make the exercise more challenging.

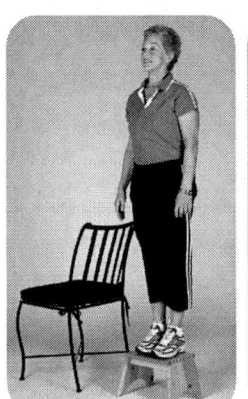

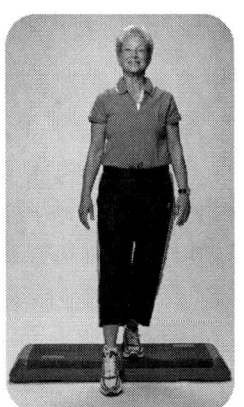

Forward Tap

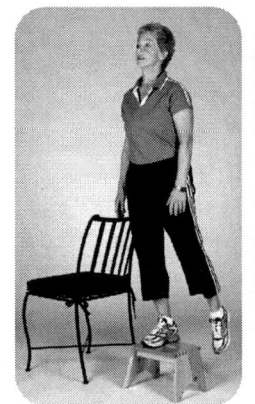

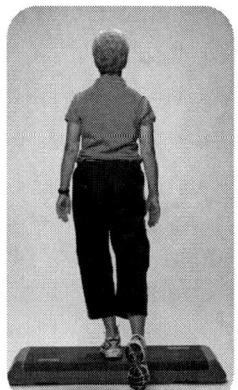

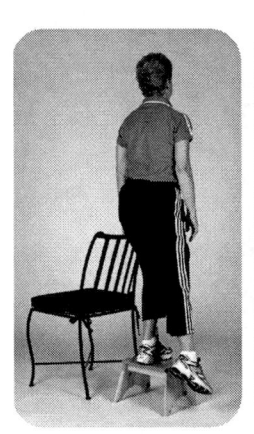

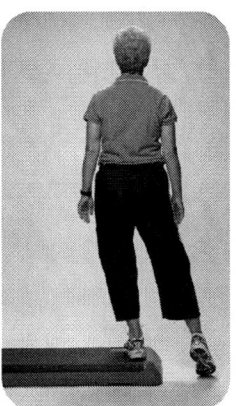

Backward Tap

Lateral Tap

Lunges

quadriceps, hamstrings, and gluteals

Positioning Stand with feet together. A support may be used for balance.

Execution Step forward with one foot and bend the knee to approximately 90 degrees of flexion. Allow the trailing knee to drop toward the floor.

Client reminder Do not allow the front knee to pass over the level of the front toes.

Modification Hold hand weights while performing the exercise.

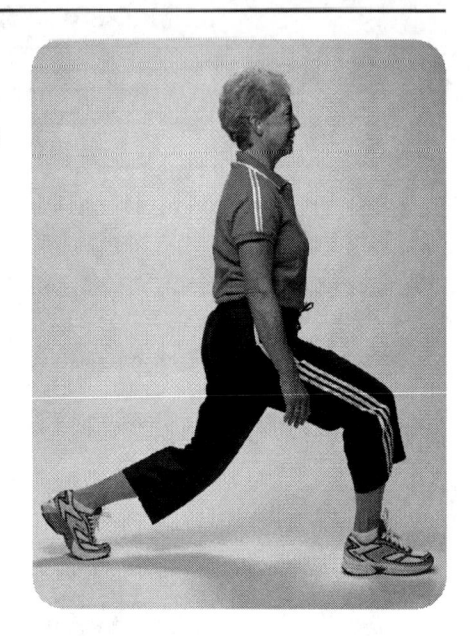

TOTAL HIP REPLACEMENT EXERCISES

The most important muscles to strengthen after a total hip replacement are the muscles that provide stability to the joint, specifically the gluteal muscles. The gluteal muscles assist with standing upright and give the hip stability during ambulation.

No matter how long ago the client underwent a total hip replacement, be aware of the hip precautions. Some physicians will allow their patients to reduce the restrictions after 3 to 6 months while others want the precautions kept in place forever. Make sure your client is aware of his or her own particular situation and, if in doubt, contact the physician. Finally, it is very important for the client following surgery to continue with some form of activity in order to maintain strength and mobility in the lower body.

Beginner Exercises

These exercises are for clients who are deconditioned or still have moderate hip and gluteal weakness.

Quadriceps Push · quadriceps

The quadriceps muscle group is made up of the rectus femoris, vastus lateralis, vastus intermedius, and vastus medialis.

Positioning Sit on a mat or lie on the back with the involved leg straight.

Execution Push the back of the knee down toward the mat, attempting to straighten the leg as much as possible. Hold for 5 seconds.

Client reminder Tighten the muscle on the front of the thigh.

Common error Using the buttocks instead of the quadriceps to push the leg down.

Modification A small rolled towel can be placed underneath the knee if the straightened position of the leg is uncomfortable.

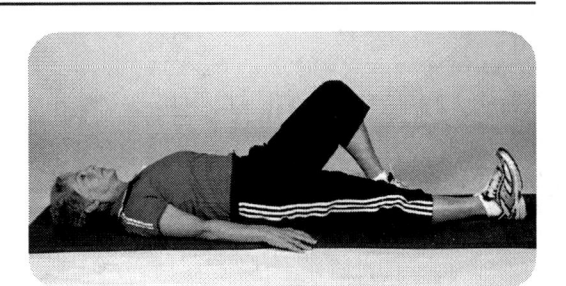

Straight Leg Lift · quadriceps and iliopsoas

Positioning Lie flat or propped on the elbows with the involved leg straight. Bend the opposite knee.

Execution Keeping the knee straight, lift the leg approximately 12 inches off the mat. Hold for 5 seconds.

Client reminder Keep the leg straight.

Common error Allowing the knee to bend and lifting primarily with the hip flexors.

Modification Add weights close to the knee at first then place them closer to the ankle to make the exercise more challenging.

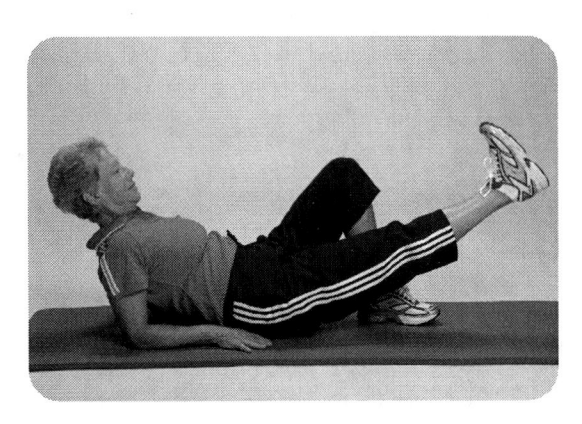

Straight Leg Lift with Toe Out   quadriceps, especially the vastus medialis, and iliopsoas

Positioning Lie flat or propped on the elbows. With the opposite leg bent, straighten the involved leg and turn the toe outward.

Execution Keeping the knee straight lift the leg approximately 12 inches off the mat. Hold for 5 seconds.

Client reminder Keep the leg straight.

Common error Allowing the knee to bend and lifting primarily with the hip flexors.

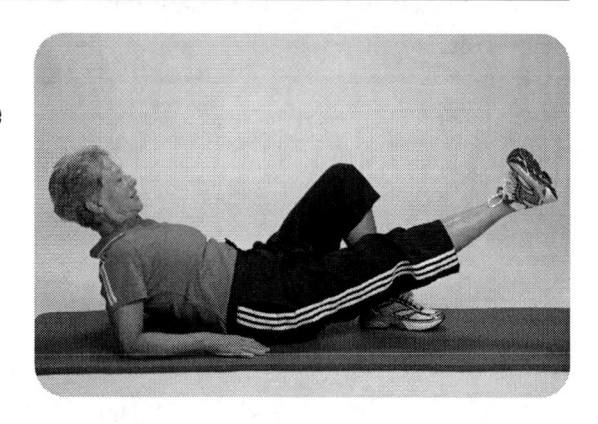

Modification Add weights close to the knee at first then place them closer to the ankle to make the exercise more challenging.

Leg Kick-Out   quadriceps

Positioning Sit on a table, bench, or chair.

Execution Straighten the knee fully and hold for 5 seconds.

Client reminder Keep the thigh supported.

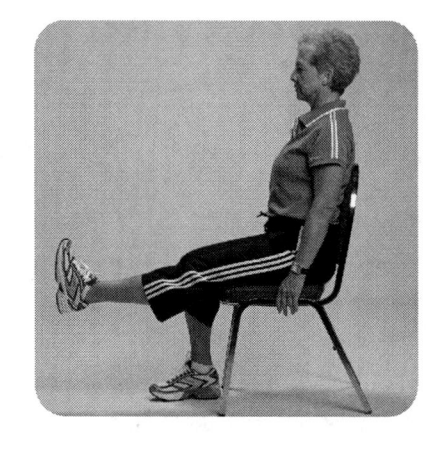

Modification Add weights close to the knee at first then place them closer to the ankle to make the exercise more challenging.

Gluteus Squeeze

gluteus maximus

Positioning Lie on the back with legs straight or bent.

Execution Squeeze buttocks together and hold for 5 seconds.

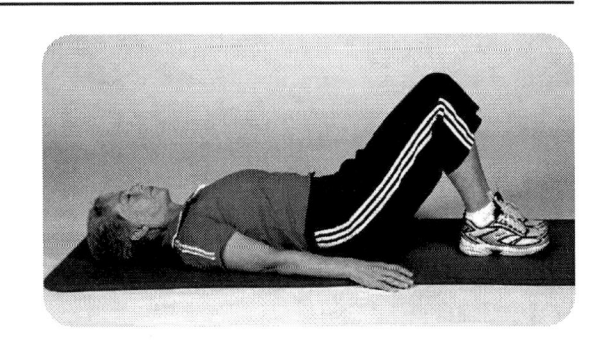

Heel Dig

hamstring

Positioning Lie on the back with the involved leg bent and heel on the mat.

Execution Push heel down into the mat and hold for 5 seconds.

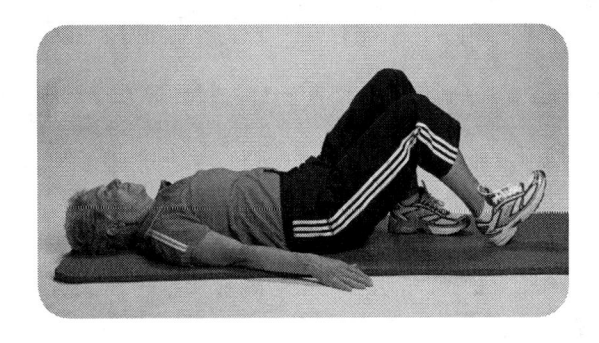

Pillow Squeeze

hip adductor group

Positioning Lie on the back with both knees bent and feet flat. Place a folded pillow between the knees.

Execution Squeeze pillow between knees and hold for 5 seconds.

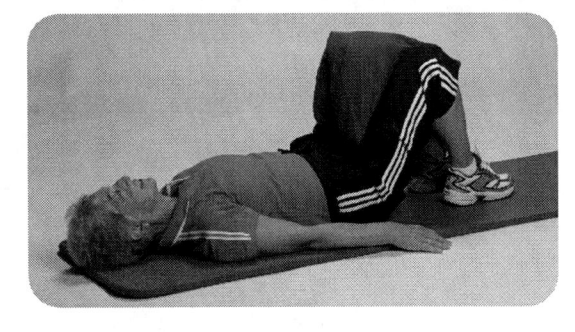

Flexibility Exercises

Flexibility exercises for the client with a total hip replacement are not as essential as for the total knee replacement client. Stretching following a total hip replacement should be performed judiciously and in accordance with the hip precautions. Although no specific time frame exists for beginning stretching exercises, it is important to remember that the hip is relatively unstable for a few months.

Anterior Hip Stretch — iliopsoas and quadriceps

This stretch can be used if the client has tightness in the anterior hip from prolonged ambulation with a forward flexed trunk to protect the hip.

Positioning Lie on back with a folded towel or pillow under the buttock of the involved side.

Execution Stay in this position for 3–5 minutes with a stretch being felt in the front of the hip.

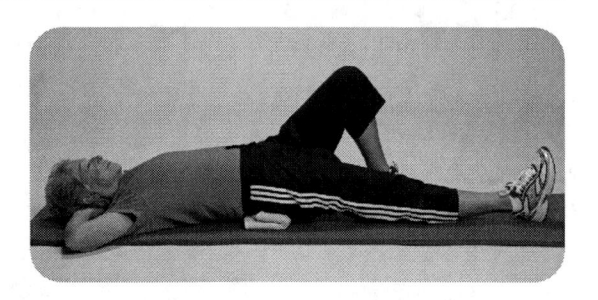

Calf Stretch — gastrocnemius

Positioning Place both hands against a wall for support with one foot behind the other.

Execution Bend the front knee toward the wall and keep the back knee straight. Hold for 20–30 seconds. Repeat 3–5 times.

Client reminder Press the back heel into the floor.

Common error Feet too far apart. Allowing the back heel to lift off the floor.

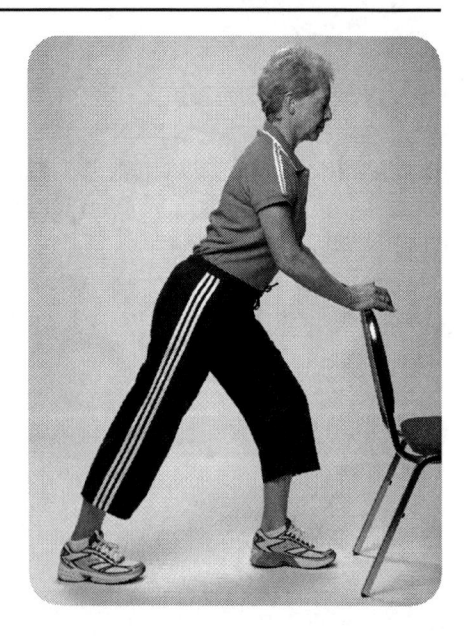

Calf Stretch on Step   **gastrocnemius**

Positioning Stand on stool or step. A support can be used for balance. Bring one heel off the edge of the step.

Execution Drop the heel below the step keeping the knee straight. Bend the knee that is standing on step. Hold for 20–30 seconds. Repeat 3–5 times.

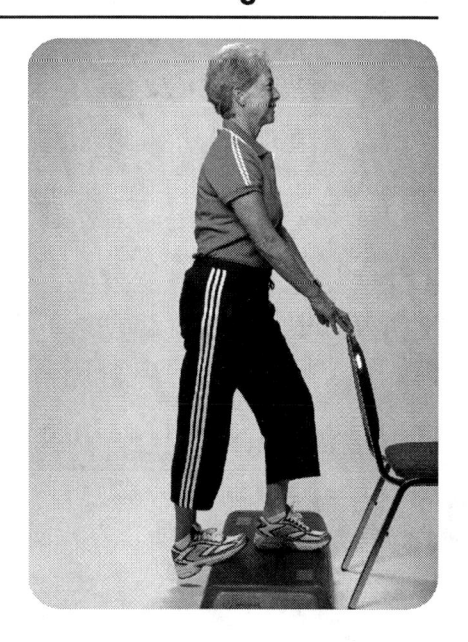

Standing Hamstring Stretch   **medial and lateral hamstrings**

Positioning Standing, prop one heel on a stool or step.

Execution Lean forward at the waist with the trunk straight. Hold 20–30 seconds. Repeat 3–5 times.

Client reminder Keep the back flat and the knee straight.

Common errors Rounding the back. Putting the foot flat on the stool.

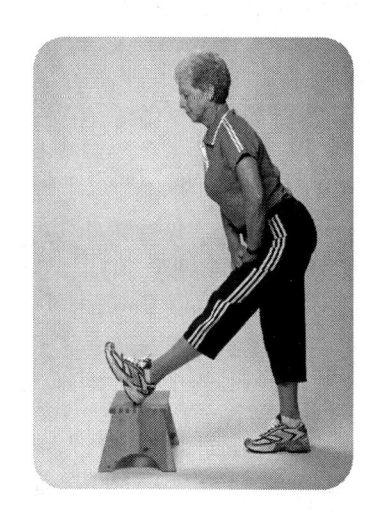

Cardiovascular Endurance

Recumbent Bicycle

Positioning Each knee should have a slight bend when the leg is at the most extended position.

Treadmill

Begin without an incline. The treadmill can also be used to reinforce proper gait pattern with slow walking.

Elliptical and Stair Stepper

The elliptical and stair stepper exercises would only be appropriate for the very advanced clients who have good quadriceps strength, hip stability, balance, and well-trained cardiovascular endurance.

Intermediate Exercises

These exercises are for clients who are able to perform the beginner exercises with little to no difficulty and are working to improve their lower-body strength.

Sidelying Abduction — **quadriceps, especially the vastus lateralis, gluteus medius and minimus**

Positioning Lie with the involved leg or surgical leg on the top. Lower leg is bent at the knee. Keep pillow separating legs so involved side does not cross over the midline.

Execution Keeping the knee straight, lift the leg toward the ceiling.

Client reminder Keep the body and knee straight.

Modification Add weights close to the knee at first then place them closer to the ankle to make the exercise more challenging.

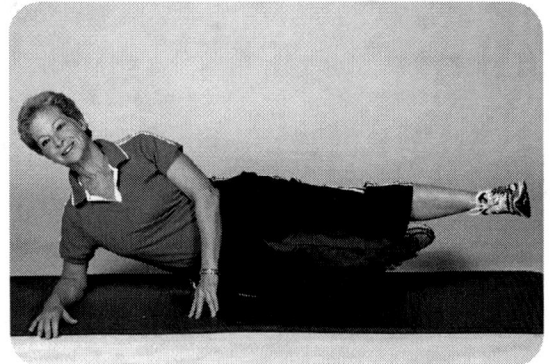

Resisted-Band Leg Pulls

Positioning Stand with the resisted band around the ankle and the other portion of the band attached to something sturdy. Use a support for balance if needed.

Execution This exercise can be performed in four different directions: hip flexion, hip extension, hip abduction, and hip adduction.

Client reminders Perform exercises in a slow and controlled manner. Stand up straight and do not lean forward or to the side. Keep knee of active leg straight but not locked.

Common errors Bending the knee of the active leg. Leaning forward as pulling band back.

Modification Increase the resistance of the band.

Note The client will often feel a greater strain on the leg they are standing on than the leg they are pulling the band with. The progression would be: (1) involved leg pulling the band and (2) standing on the involved leg and pulling the band with the other side.

Flexion   quadriceps and iliopsoas

Execution Pull band forward, keeping the knee straight.

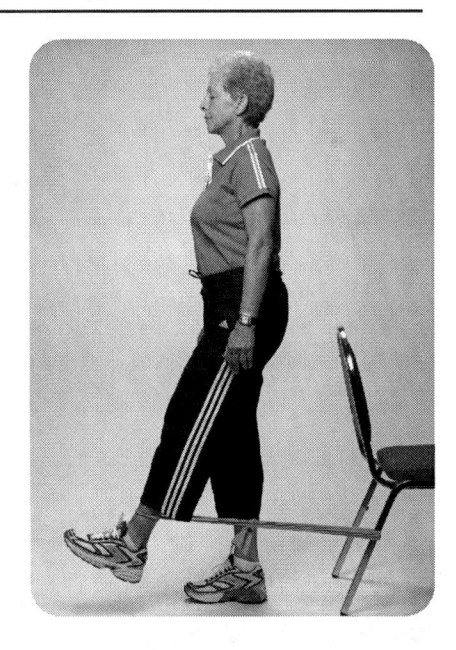

Extension quadriceps, gluteus maximus, and hamstrings

Execution Pull band backward, keeping the knee straight.

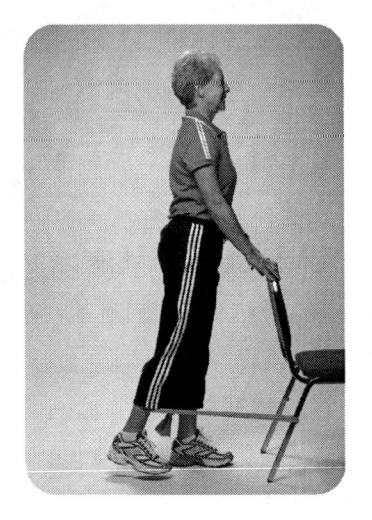

Abduction quadriceps, especially the vastus lateralis, gluteus medius, and minimus

Execution Pull band out to the side, keeping the knee straight.

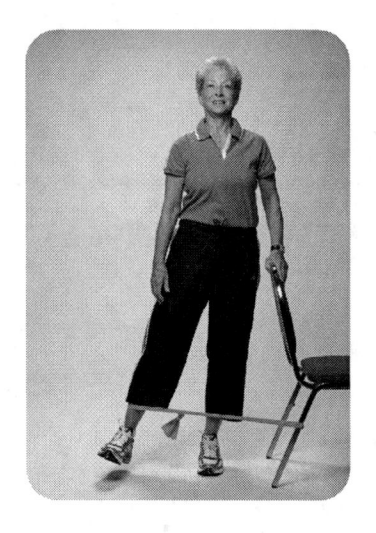

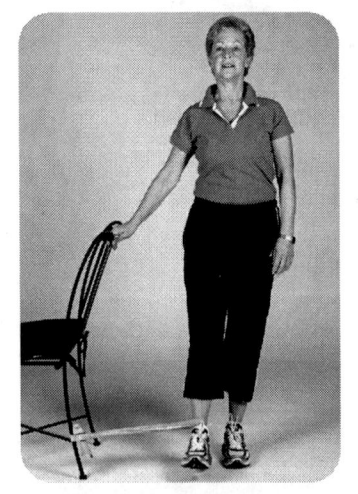

Adduction quadriceps, especially the vastus medialis, adductor group, and gracilis

Execution Pull band in toward midline, but **do not** cross the midline, keeping knee straight.

"Clams"
gluteus medius and minimus

Positioning Lie with the involved leg on top. Place a pillow between the knees so the upper leg will not cross the midline of the body. Bend both knees and keep the ankles touching each other.

Execution Carefully lift the top knee off the bottom one, keeping feet together and trunk straight.

Client reminders Do not let feet separate. Keep trunk straight.

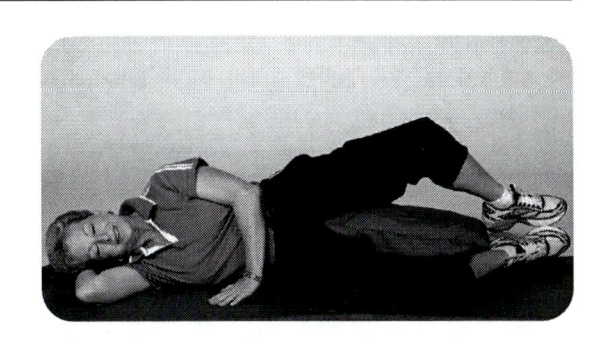

Knee Separation
gluteus medius and minimus

Positioning Lie on the back with both knees bent and feet flat. Wrap a resisted band around the thighs.

Execution Separate knees and pull against the resistance of the band.

Client reminder Perform exercise in a slow and controlled manner.

Modification Increase resistance of the band.

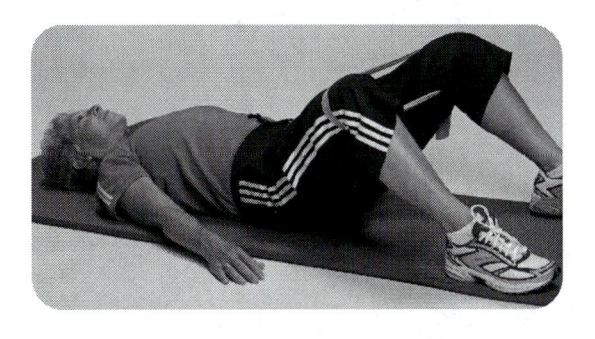

Bridging
gluteus maximus and hamstrings

Positioning Lie on the back with both knees bent and feet flat.

Execution Lift the hips and try not to let the buttocks sink. The shoulders, hips, and knees should be aligned.

Client reminders Keep hips lifted and try not to sink down.

Modifications While holding the bridge position, perform the knee separation exercise. While holding the bridge position, perform the pillow squeeze exercise.

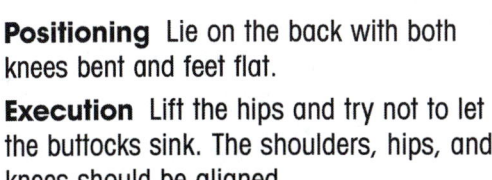

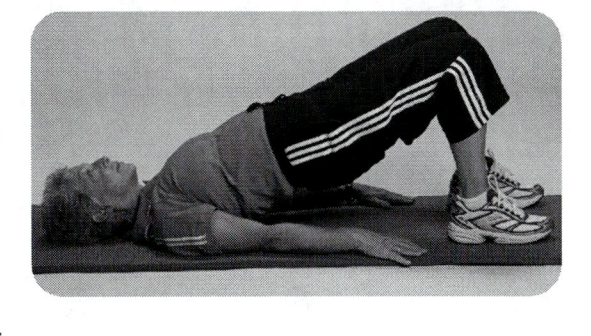

Wall Squats

quadriceps and gluteals

Positioning Rest the back on a wall with both feet approximately 2–3 feet from the wall. Make sure the knees are not farther out than the toes.

Execution Slide the back down the wall and hold for 5 seconds. Straighten both knees and slide back to starting position.

Client reminders Keep knees from going over toes.

Modifications Use an inflatable ball behind the small of the back when sliding down the wall. Sit and hold the squat for 10–30 seconds.

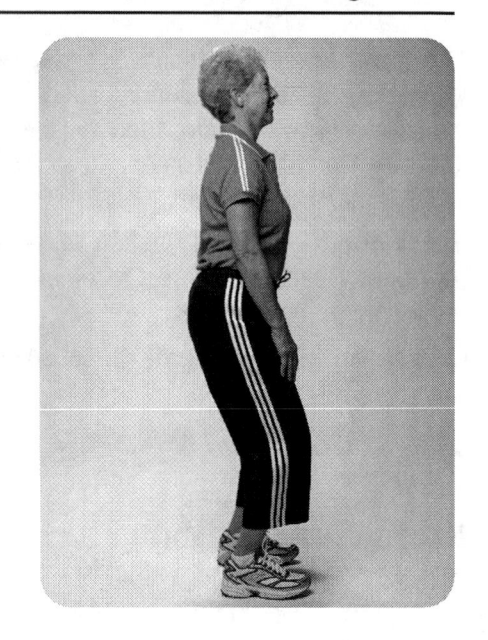

Steps*

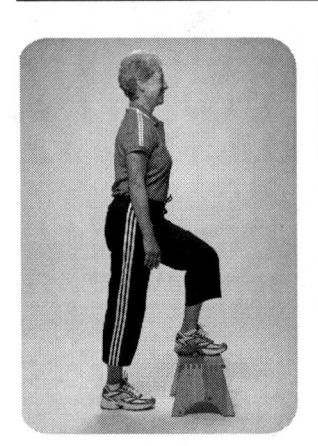

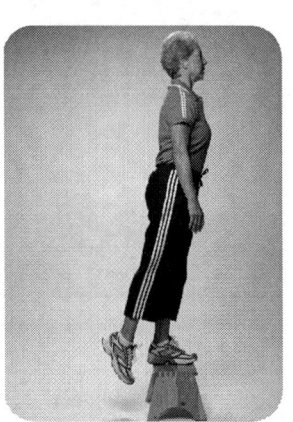

Forward   **quadriceps**

Execution Facing the stool, step up with the involved leg.

Modification Increase the step height.

*Hold onto a support for balance if needed when performing step exercises.

Backward
quadriceps, gluteals, and hamstrings

Execution Standing on the stool, step down onto the floor, keeping the involved leg on the stool. Step back onto the stool.

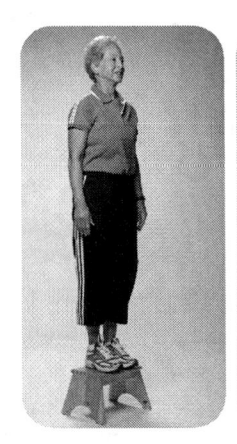

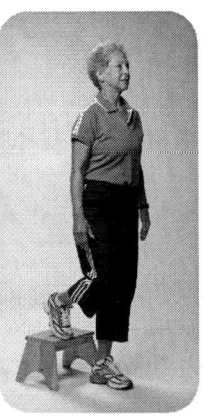

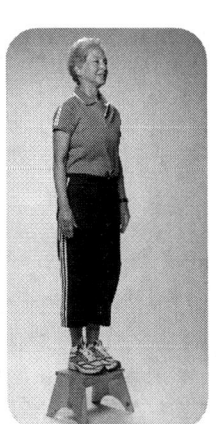

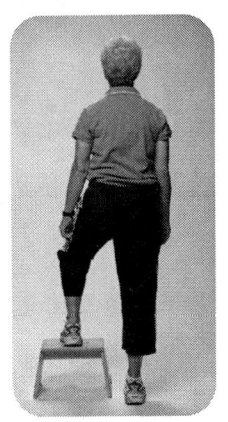

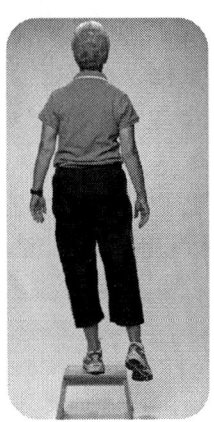

Lateral
quadriceps, especially the vastus lateralis, gluteus medius, and minimus

Execution Standing with the stool next to the involved leg, step sideways onto the stool.

Hip Extension on Hands and Knees   gluteals and hamstrings

Positioning On hands and knees.

Execution Extend the knee and lift the leg to a position that is level with the trunk.

Client reminders Keep the abdominals tight and the leg level. Do not arch the back.

Modification Add ankle weights.

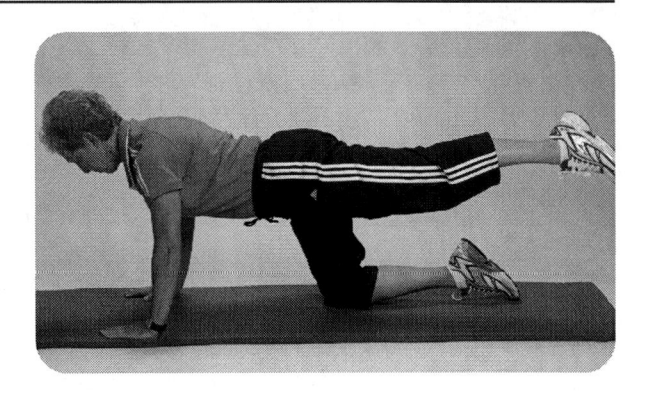

Advanced Exercises

Hip Resistance Machine   **hip flexor, extensor, abductor, and adductor muscle groups, knee flexor and extensor groups**

Although this machine emphasizes hip motion, knee strength is required to stabilize on the stationary, or standing, leg. For example, if the client has had a left total knee replacement, he or she may be more challenged by standing on the left leg while performing the exercises with the right leg.

Because each machine is slightly different, a full explanation of the execution of the exercise will not be given. Keep in mind that the exercises can be performed in four different directions of the hip, including flexion, extension, abduction, and adduction.

Leg Press   **quadriceps and gluteus maximus**

Positioning Lie face up on the "sled" with feet on the foot plate. Hip flexion should be less than 90 degrees in the start position.

Execution Push the sled away as the feet remain stationary.

Modification The reverse motion is possible with other types of machines where the plate is pushed away and the body remains stationary.

Knee Extension Machine   **quadriceps**

Positioning Seated with the bar over the shins.

Execution Straighten knees without locking them.

Note This exercise should **not** be performed with the involved leg only because it places a great deal of torque through the knee joint.

Bridging on Ball

gluteals and hamstrings

Positioning Lie on the back with lower legs and feet resting on the ball.

Execution Lift buttocks off the mat and straighten legs.

Common errors Lifting the buttocks only part way off the mat. Pushing down with the arms

Modification Placing the ball farther away from the body will increase the challenge.

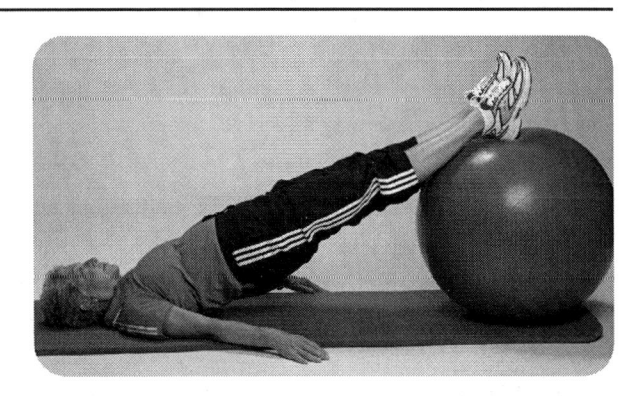

Bridging Kick-Out

gluteals, hamstrings, and quadriceps

Positioning Lie on the back with the knees bent and feet flat.

Execution Lift buttocks off mat. While holding the raised position, straighten one leg. Return to the starting position and repeat on the opposite leg.

Client reminder Keep buttocks lifted the entire time.

Common errors Lifting buttocks only partially off the mat. Dropping pelvis on side of side of lifted leg.

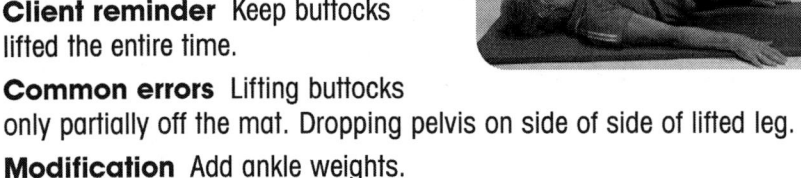

Modification Add ankle weights.

Bridging March

gluteals, hamstrings, and iliopsoas

Positioning Lie on back with knees bent and feet flat.

Execution Lift buttocks off mat. While holding the raised position, lift one foot slightly off the mat. Alternate feet.

Client reminder Keep buttocks lifted the entire time.

Common errors Lifting buttocks only partially off the mat. Dropping pelvis on side of side of lifted leg.

Modification Add ankle weights.

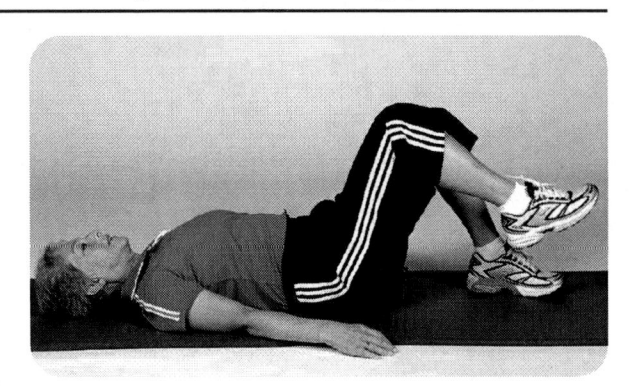

Step Taps* requires good eccentric muscle control of the quadriceps, hip stability strength, and gastrocnemius flexibility

Positioning Stand on a stool or small step. These exercises should be performed holding onto a support for balance.

Execution While standing on the involved leg, squat slightly until the toe of the opposite leg is touching the ground. Immediately straighten the support leg on the step so weight is not placed on the foot tapping the ground.

Client reminder Place only the toe down to tap the floor.

Modification Increase the height of the step to make the exercise more challenging.

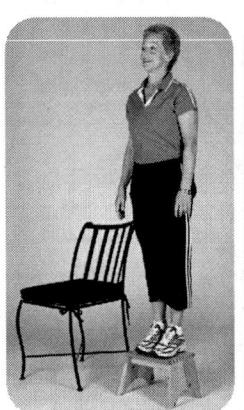

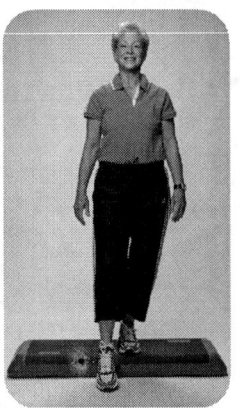

Forward Tap

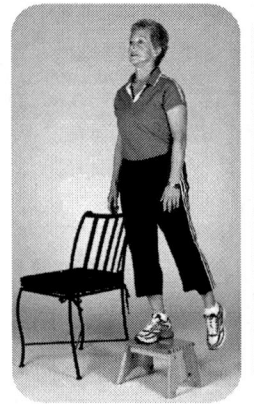

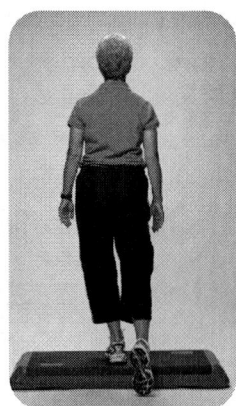

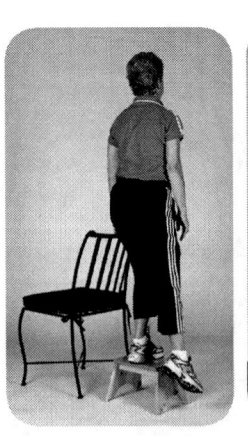

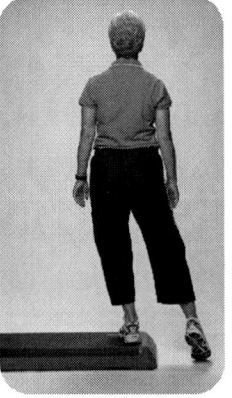

Backward Tap

Lateral Tap

*Hold onto a support for balance if needed when performing step exercises.

Lunges   quadriceps, hamstrings, and gluteals

Positioning Stand with feet together. A support can be used for balance.

Execution Step forward with one foot and bend the knee to approximately 90 degrees of flexion. Allow the trailing knee to drop toward the floor.

Client reminder Do not allow the front knee to pass over the level of the front toes.

Modification Hold hand weights while performing the exercise.

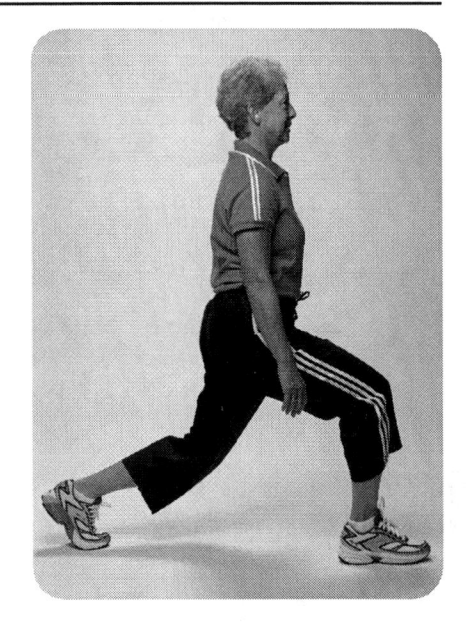

Study Questions

Complete the following questions. The answer key is on page 86.

1. True or false. The Straight Leg Lift with Toe Out works on the strength of the quadriceps, specifically the vastus medialis.

2. True or false:. It is important to start all total joint replacement clients with the beginner exercises.

3. Name the two muscles that are strengthened when performing the Knee Separation exercise.

    (1) _____

    (2) _____

4. True or false. One way in which to modify the Step exercise is to increase the height of the step.

5. True or false. Bridging Kick Out is an example of an intermediate total hip replacement exercise because it does not involve the client standing.

6. Which muscle is usually in a protective flexed posture after a knee replacement surgery?

    _____

7. True or false. Hip precautions apply only to static positions like sitting or standing and do not need to be followed when using the machines.

8. Which exercise requires good eccentric control of the quadriceps muscle?

    _____

CHAPTER 5

Case Studies

Total Knee Replacement

Background Information

A 67-year-old male client comes to see you having had a left total knee replacement approximately 2 months ago. Mr. Green's rehabilitation history includes a 3-day stay in the hospital followed by 2 weeks at an inpatient rehabilitation center where he worked on walking with a cane and increasing his knee range of motion. Mr. Green did not have home health or outpatient physical therapy but he continued to work on the exercises that his physical therapist gave him in the rehab center. Mr. Green states that he saw his doctor about 2 weeks ago and was told he was progressing well as he no longer requires the use of his cane. The doctor encouraged Mr. Green to pursue working with a personal trainer to improve his strength, endurance, and stamina. Mr. Green's goal is to return to playing golf with his wife and playing with his grandchildren.

Mr. Green's past medical history includes a heart bypass operation approximately 7 years ago. He has been healthy ever since. Mr. Green currently takes a beta blocker for his heart, blood pressure medication, and a pill to lower his cholesterol. He does not use nitroglycerin.

When you test Mr. Green's strength, you notice a deficit in the left quadriceps as well as the left hamstrings. His left knee extension range of motion is -25 degrees and knee flexion is 115 degrees. The left quadriceps is ¾ inch smaller than the right, measured 5 inches above the knee. During the single-leg stance, Mr. Green was able to stand on his left leg for 4 seconds and his right leg for 8 seconds. Mr. Green walks with a slight limp on the left side but does not use a cane.

Goals

The client will work toward achieving the following goals within 2 to 3 months:

- Improve the strength of the left knee.
- Increase the muscle girth around the left thigh.
- Eliminate the client's limp while walking.
- Maximize the range of motion of the left knee.
- Return the client to golfing activity as allowed by the physician.

Exercise Routine

This exercise routine should be performed 3 times a week. Begin the workout session with cardiovascular conditioning to increase circulation as well as to increase the flexibility of the knee. The best mode of exercise is the stationary bike so he can work on his knee range of motion at the same time as his cardiovascular conditioning. The bike should be ridden from 10 to 20 minutes depending on the client's current cardiovascular conditioning level.

Flexibility exercises should be performed following cardiovascular training. All muscle groups are appropriate to stretch, especially the hamstrings. The hamstrings can be stretched either in the supine, prone, or standing position to increase knee extension. The heel to buttocks stretch for quadriceps flexibility would help increase the decreased knee flexion range of motion. The gastrocnemius stretch on the step is a good idea as the client continues to have a slight limp. Abnormal ambulation is usually accompanied by inflexible lower extremity musculature, especially the gastrocnemius muscle.

Strengthening the lower extremity follows the stretching exercises. The following exercises are just a few of the exercises that would be appropriate to address the client's strength deficits, single-leg stance time, and girth measurement.

- Straight Leg Raise
- Straight Leg Raise with Toe Out
- Knee Extension Machine
- Leg Press
- Steps: Forward, Lateral, Backward
- Sideways Walking with Elastic Band
- Resisted-Band Leg Pulls

Exercise Progression

In general, these exercises can be progressed as follows:

- Start with low resistance and low repetitions (2 sets of 10).
- Increase repetitions first, then increase resistance.
- If necessary, decrease the repetitions when the resistance is increased.

Monitor the client's heart rate, pain level, and perceived exertion during the course of workout. For motivational purposes you can remind the client how each exercise can improve his golf game.

Total Hip Replacement

Background Information

Mrs. Riley is a 52-year-old female who was referred to you by a physical therapist for continued strengthening after a right total hip replacement 5 months ago. She was involved in a severe car accident where she sustained a compound fracture of her femur and a stress fracture to her acetabulum. The surgical team decided to perform a total hip replacement due to the extensive damage. She was in the acute care hospital for 1 month, a rehabilitation hospital for 2 months, and just finished outpatient therapy 2 weeks ago. She has no past medical history and takes pain medication only when needed. Although Mrs. Riley still uses a cane when walking, she can't wait until she can start walking again in the mornings with her neighbors. At this time Mrs. Riley's doctor wants her to continue following the hip precautions.

With muscle testing you find that she has a very weak gluteus medius and gluteus maximus muscle. Her lower body has full range of motion and flexibility, but her quadriceps exhibit continued weakness. She is unable to perform the single-leg stance on the right leg at all.

Goals

The client will work toward achieving the following goals in 3 to 4 months.

- Improve the right quadriceps strength.
- Improve gluteus medius and maximus strength of the right hip to improve her single-leg stance time and stability of the hip.
- Increase ambulation tolerance on the treadmill to enable her to return to walking with her neighbors.
- Improve overall strength, balance, and flexibility so that she will have decreased dependence on her walking cane.

Exercise Routine

Begin the workout session with cardiovascular conditioning to increase circulation and improve the flexibility of the lower extremity. Mrs. Riley could either ride the stationary bike or walk on the treadmill, as long as the hip precautions are followed when riding the bike. Time on the treadmill should be progressed according to her walking goals. Mrs. Riley should use the rails on the treadmill to encourage ambulation without an assistive device.

Flexibility of the gastrocnemius is the only real stretch that is beneficial for Mrs. Riley to perform at this time. She can perform this stretch either on the step or against the wall.

Strengthening exercises for the muscles surrounding the hip are the most important. Mrs. Riley's gluteal muscles exhibit the greatest weakness; therefore, the most appropriate exercises would be:

- "Clams"
- Sidelying Abduction
- Knee Separation

As she progresses, bridging exercises including Bridging on Ball, Bridging Kick-Out, and Bridging March can be used for a greater challenge. As her endurance and gait pattern improve, duration on the treadmill should be increased so that she can work toward her goal of walking with her neighbors without the use of her cane.

Exercise Progression

These exercises can be progressed as follows:

- Start with low resistance and low repetitions (2 sets of 10).
- Increase repetitions first, then resistance.
- If necessary, decrease the repetitions when the resistance is increased.

Monitor the client's heart rate, pain level, and perceived exertion during the course of the workout. For motivational purposes you can remind the client how each exercise helps her to get one "step" closer to walking with her friends again.

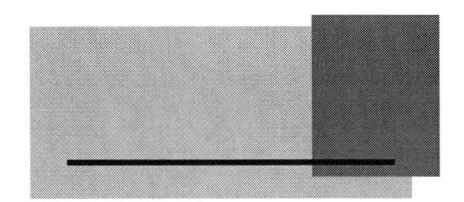

Answer Keys

Chapter 1

1. Improve function and decrease pain.
2. True.
3. Pain in the joint, pain that is progressive in nature, stiffness in joint, limitations in joint movement, swelling around the joint, and crunching or creaking sounds with joint movement.
4. True.
5. True.
6. Osteoarthritis, rheumatoid arthritis, post-traumatic arthritis, hip fracture, and hip necrosis.
7. Severe pain, pain during rest, chronic swelling, deformity or stiffness, inadequate pain relief with medications, and failure to improve with other types of treatments.
8. Stem, ball, and socket
9. False.
10. True.
11. Decreased bleeding from the incision, decreased trauma to the muscles and tendons, decreased pain and improved rehabilitation capacity.

Chapter 2

1. Obesity, diabetes, and hypertension.
2. Limit hip bend to 90 degrees, do not cross the leg past midline of the body, and do not turn the leg too far inward or outward.

3. *Safe:* low-impact activity such as: walking, swimming, golfing (with spikeless shoes and a cart, bicycling (on level surfaces), stationary bike riding, and ballroom dancing.
   Unsafe: jogging, skiing, horseback riding, high-impact aerobics, contact sports, and tennis and other racquet sports.
4. True.

Chapter 3

1. False.
2. False.
3. When was your surgery? What specific type of surgery did you undergo? Is your prosthesis cemented or noncemented? What type of rehabilitation did you have after being discharged from the hospital? When was your last visit to the orthopedic surgeon? When was the last time you worked with a physical therapist, and where was it? (at the hospital, at home, or as an outpatient) Have you been performing any type of exercise at home? Has the physician given you any specific restrictions? Are you still observing the hip precautions? Do you know what the hip precautions are?
4. Heart rate, perceived exertion, pain scale, and physical observation.
5. False.
6. Single-leg Stance.

Chapter 4

1. True.
2. False.
3. Gluteus medius and gluteus minimus.
4. True.
5. False.
6. Hamstring.
7. False.
8. Step taps.

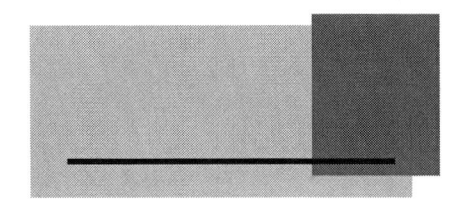

References

American Academy of Orthopedic Surgeons. Total Joint Replacement. http://orthoinfo.aaos.org (accessed November 16, 2005).

———. Total Knee Replacement. http://orthoinfo.aaos.org (accessed November 16, 2005).

———. Activities after a Hip Replacement. http://orthoinfo.aaos.org (accessed December 19, 2005).

———. Total Hip Replacement. http://orthoinfo.aaos.org (accessed December 19, 2005).

———. Cemented and Cementless Knee Replacement. http://orthoinfo.aaos.org (accessed January 4, 2006).

———. Knee Implants. http://orthoinfo.aaos.org (accessed January 4, 2006).

———. Minimally Invasive Hip Replacement. http://orthoinfo.aaos.org (accessed January 4, 2006).

———. Minimally Invasive Total Knee. Replacement. http://orthoinfo.aaos.org (accessed January 4, 2006).

———. Hip Implants. http://orthoinfo.aaos.org (accessed December 19, 2006).

Arthritis Foundation. How Do You Know It's Time for Surgery? www.arthritis.org/conditions/SurgeryCenter/when_surgery.asp (accessed December 15, 2005).

Bren, Linda. 2004. Joint Replacement: An Inside Look. *FDA Consumer Magazine.* March–April. Pub No. FDA 1335C. www.fda.gov/fdac/features/2004/204_joints.html. (accessed November 16, 2005).

Encyclopedia of Surgery. Arthroplasty. www.surgeryencyclopedia.com/A-Ce/Arthroplasty.html (accessed January 23, 2006).

The Hip and Knee Institute. Long Term Care of Your Knee Replacement. www.hipsandknees.com/hip/hipcare.htm (accessed February 2, 2006).

———. Hip Implant Designs and Materials. www.hipsandknees.com/hip/hipimplants.htm (accessed February 2, 2006).

———. Total Knee Replacement Surgery. www.hipsandknees.com/knee/totalkneereplacement.htm (accessed February 2, 2006).

Joint Replacement Institute. Hip Replacement Surgery: Types and Methods of Fixation. www.jri-oh.com/hipsurgery/hip_types.asp (accessed November 16, 2005).

Kendall, F., E. McCreary, and P. Provance. 1993. *Muscles: Testing and Function.* Baltimore: Williams and Wilkins.

McGrory, Brian. Contemporary Total Hip Replacements: How Long Will They Last? www.orthoassociates.com/Totalhip1.htm (accessed February 21, 2006).

MedicineNet.com. Osteoarthritis (Degenerative Arthritis). www.medicinenet.com/osteoarthritis/article.htm (accessed on December 15, 2005).

Merritt, Richard. 2005. Diabetes, hypertension and obesity negatively effect joint replacement outcomes. *Medical News Today,* June 1. www.medicalnewstoday.com/medicalnews.php?newsid=25417 (accessed February 21, 2006).

Mizner, R., S. Petterson, J. Stevens, K Vandenborne, and L. Snyder-Mackler. 2005. Early Quadriceps Strength Loss After Total Knee Arthroplasty: The Contributions of Muscle Atrophy and Failure of Voluntary Muscle Activation. *The Journal of Bone and Joint Surgery* 87, no. 5: 1047–1053.

Orthopedics.com. Rotating Knee Replacements. http://orthopedics.about.com/od/hipreplacement /a/rotating.htm (accessed January 1, 2006).

Total Hip Replacement.net. Surgical Approaches: Anterolateral. www.totalhipreplacement.net/THR/surgery/surgical_approaches/anterolateral_medical.htm (accessed March 1, 2006).

———. Surgical Approaches: Posterior. www.totalhipreplacement.net/THR/surgery/surgical_approaches/posterior_medical.htm. (accessed March 1, 2006).

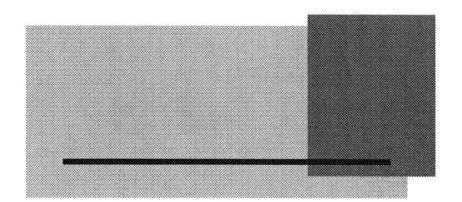

About the Author

Erin Erb Roblero, MSPT, C-PT, graduated summa cum laude from Boston University in 1996 with a bachelor's of science degree in health studies. In 1998 she completed her master's of science degree in physical therapy from the same university. Since that time she has been a practicing physical therapist in Virginia and now in Texas. Erin has worked with a variety of patient populations in numerous settings, including home healthcare, hospital acute care, and outpatient orthopedics. Within these settings, she has worked with hundreds of patients who have undergone a total joint replacement.

Erin has been certified as a personal trainer through the National Strength and Conditioning Association since 2000. In 2002 Erin joined the Desert Southwest Fitness team of course reviewers and has participated in the development of three courses. Erin has authored six articles over the past two years for *Advance for Physical Therapists and PTAs*. This is the second course Erin has written for Desert Southwest Fitness. Foam Roller Fitness was published last year with great success. She hopes to continue her writing career while working as a physical therapist in San Antonio, Texas.